AF364248

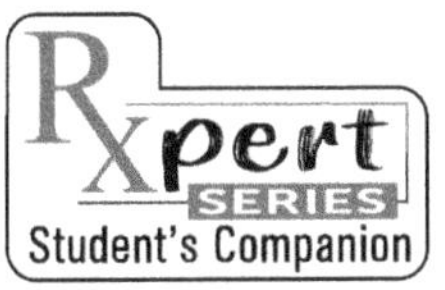

Biochemistry and Clinical Pathology

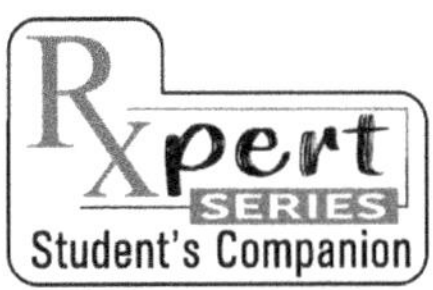

Biochemistry and Clinical Pathology

Pooja A Chawla

PhD, M Pharm
Professor and Head
Department of Pharmaceutical Chemistry and Analysis
ISF College of Pharmacy, Moga, 142001, Punjab

Simranpreet K Wahan

MSc
Assistant Professor
Department of Pharmaceutical Chemistry,
ISF College of Pharmacy, Moga

Naresh K Rangra

PhD, M Pharm
Associate Professor
Department of Pharmaceutical Chemistry,
ISF College of Pharmacy, Moga

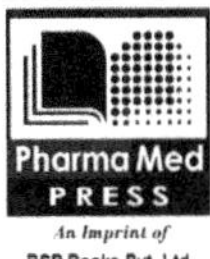

PharmaMed Press

An imprint of BSP Books Pvt. Ltd

4-4-309/316, Giriraj Lane,
Sultan Bazar, Hyderabad - 500 095.

Biochemistry and Clinical Pathology
by Pooja A Chawla, Simranpreet K Wahan and Naresh K Rangra

Published by:

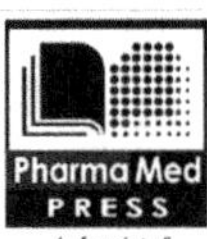

PharmaMed Press

An imprint of BSP Books Pvt. Ltd.

4-4-309/316, Giriraj Lane, Sultan Bazar, Hyderabad - 500 095.
Phone: 040-23445688; Fax: 91+40-23445611
e-mail: info@pharmamedpress.com
www.pharmamedpress.com/pharmamedpress.net

ISBN: 978-93-95039-93-2 (Hardback)

Preface

Biochemistry is an essential subject to understand the molecular basis of biomolecules and their metabolism. It helps to understand molecular basis of diseases and drug action. The pharmacokinetic profile of a drug is difficult to understand without a biochemical background. The book is written in easy-to-understand language and is well illustrated with figures for beginners of biochemistry. This book covers the syllabus prescribed by Pharmacy Council of India (PCI) for diploma students of pharmacy program. But this book will be beneficial for bachelor of pharmacy, paramedical as well medical students in understanding the basics of biochemistry.

-Authors

Contents

Chapter – 1

Introduction to Biochemistry

Chapter – 2

Carbohydrates

Chapter – 3

Proteins

Chapter – 4

Lipids

Chapter – 5

Nucleic Acids

Chapter – 6

Enzymes

Chapter – 7

Vitamins

Chapter – 8

Metabolism

Chapter – 9

Minerals

Chapter – 10

Water and Electrolytes

Chapter – 11

Introduction to Biotechnology

Chapter – 12
Organ Function Tests

Chapter – 13
Introduction to Pathology Blood and Urine

Question Bank from Previous Years' Examination 131

Chapter 1

Introduction to Biochemistry

Carl Neuberg coined the word "biochemistry" in 1903. Biochemistry is the study of the chemistry of life and living processes in general. Biochemistry is involved in every element of life, including conception, growth, reproduction, ageing, and death. Every movement of life, in fact, is filled with hundreds of biological reactions. Biochemistry is the most inventive and rapidly evolving field of medicine. This is demonstrated by the fact that biochemistry researchers have received the majority of Nobel Prizes in Medicine and Physiology over the years.

Origin of Biochemistry: the discovery that a cell-free yeast can ferment sugar-initiated biochemistry.

The discovery of yeast's capacity to transform carbohydrates to ethyl alcohol predates recorded history. This process, however, did not directly lead to the study of biochemistry until the early twentieth century. Despite extensive research into winemaking, Louis Pasteur, a prominent French scientist, maintained that fermentation was possible only in imperfect cells. The Büchner brothers, who discovered that fertilization could take place in cellular parts in 1899, pointed out his mistake. These findings are due to the storage of yeast extracted from a concentrated sugar solution plant that was added as a preservative. In the early years of the 20th century, these discoveries resulted in a rapid and very fruitful experiment that led to the study of biochemistry. This study found important functions of inorganic phosphate, ADP, ATP, and NADH, as well as phosphorylated sugars and chemical processes and enzymes that convert glucose into pyruvate or ethanol and $-CO_2$ (fermentation). After research in the 1930s and 1940s, scientists discovered the intermediate cycles of citric acid and urea biosynthesis, as well as the important roles of cofactors found in vitamins or "coenzymes" such as thiamine pyrophosphate, riboflavin, and, finally, coenzyme A, coenzyme Q, and cobamide coenzymes. The 1950s described the biosynthesis processes of pentoses and the breakdown of amino acids and lipids, as well as how complex carbohydrates are created and broken down into simple sugars.

Scope of Biochemistry in Pharmacy

For health-care practitioners, particularly physicians, learning and maintaining good health, as well as comprehending and effectively treating diseases, are two major concerns. Both of these basic difficulties are impacted by biochemistry, and the link between biochemistry and medicine is a two-way street. Many features of health and sickness have been emphasized by biochemical research, and the study of many aspects of health and disease has opened up new branches of biochemistry. Archibald Garrod, an English physician, investigated persons with the relatively unusual disorders of alkaptonuria, albinism, cystinuria, and pentosuria in the early 1900s and concluded that they were genetically determined. These are known as inborn metabolic errors, according to Garrod. His discoveries established the framework for the study of human biochemical genetics to expand. A more current example is the research of the genetic and molecular roots of familial hypercholesterolemia, a disorder that causes atherosclerosis at an early age. This enabled a broader knowledge of cell receptors and methods of absorption, not just of cholesterol, but of how other chemicals cross cell membranes, in addition to clarifying different genetic defects responsible for this sickness. The identification of oncogenes and tumour suppressor genes in cancer cells has moved emphasis to the molecular pathways that govern normal cell growth. These examples highlight how disease study may lead to new disciplines of fundamental biochemical research. Science supplies a platform for physicians and other health-care and biology professionals that impact practise, motivates curiosity, and fosters the use of scientific approaches for lifelong learning. The area of medicine will have a logical basis capable of tolerating and responding to new findings as long as medical treatment is firmly established in biochemistry and other fundamental sciences (Figure 1.1). Nutrition and Preventive Medicine are touched by biochemical research. Health is described by the World Health Organization (WHO) as a condition of "complete physical, mental, and social well-being." A healthy diet must include a range of chemicals, the most essential of which being vitamins and particular amino acids as well as fatty acids, minerals, and water. Nutrition is strongly reliant on biochemical knowledge, and biochemistry and nutrition have a number of similarities.

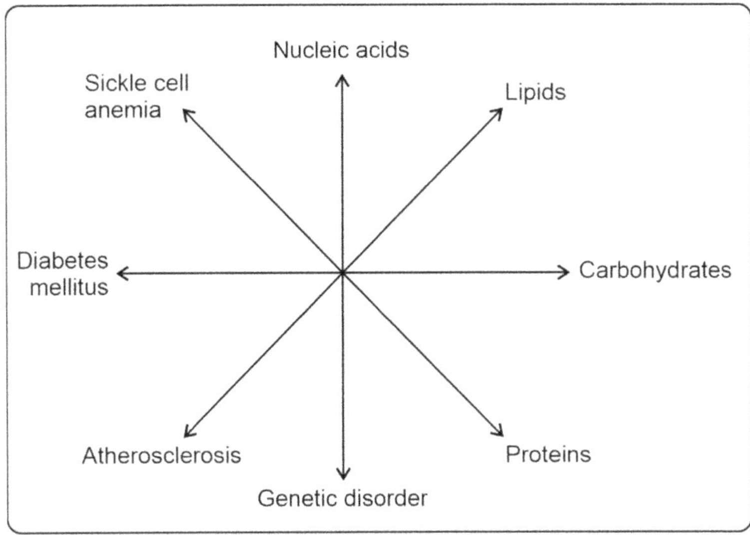

Fig. 1.1 Two-way connection of biochemistry and medicine.

Life is made up of lifeless molecules. The bacteria *Escherichia coli* has roughly 6,000 distinct chemical molecules in a single cell. Only a fraction of the 100,000 distinct kinds of molecules believed to exist in man have been identified.

Cell

Life's structural and functional unit is the cell. It can also be looked as the fundamental unit of biological activity. The contributions of Schleiden and Schwann gave rise to the idea of cell (1838). The complexity of cell structure, however, were not revealed until around 1940.

Prokaryotic and Eukaryotic Cells

The living kingdom's cells may be classified into two groups.

1. **Prokaryotes** (Greek: pro – before; karyon – nucleus) have a simple structure and lack a well-defined nucleus. Various bacteria are among them.

2. **Eukaryotes** (Greek: eu – true; karyon – nucleus) have a well-defined nucleus and more complicated structure and function than prokaryotes. Eukaryotic cells make up the higher creatures (animals and plants).

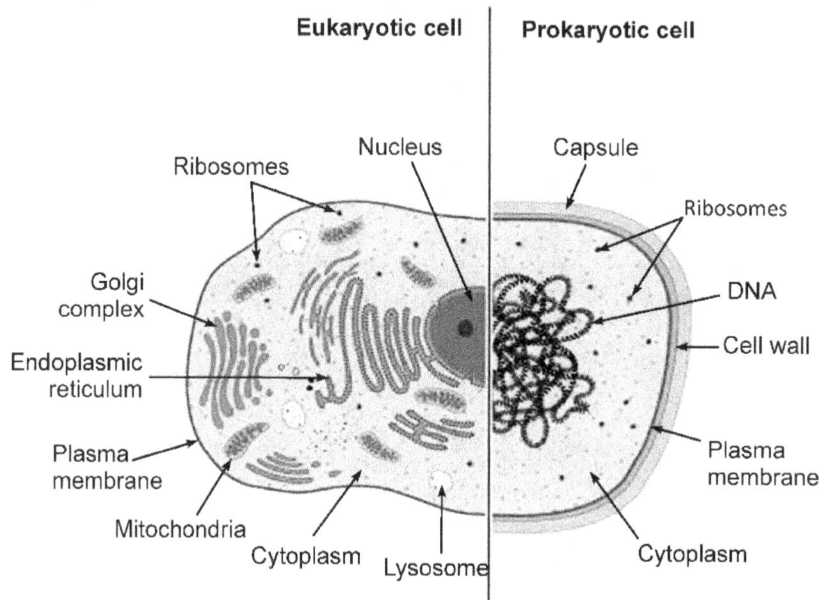

Fig. 1.2 Diagram of prokaryotic and eurkaryotic cells.

The differences between the two are shown in **Table 1.1**

Table 1.1 Differences between prokaryotic and eurkaryotic cells.

Characteristic	Prokaryotes	Eukaryotes
Size	The size is usually small (generally 1–10 µm).	The size of the cell is larger compared to prokaryotes (generally 10–100 µm).
Cell membrane	A stiff and strong cell wall surrounds the cell.	A flexible plasma membrane surrounds the cell.
Nucleus	Histones are not present; however, DNA is found as a nucleoid.	DNA is associated with histones, and the nucleus is highly defined and enclosed by a membrane.
Subcellular organelles	Absent	Organelles (mitochondria, nucleus, and lysosomes) are present inside the cell.
Energy metabolism	Mitochondria is absent and energy metabolism enzymes are linked to the membrane.	Energy-metabolizing enzymes are found in mitochondria
Cytoplasm	Organelles and cytoskeleton are absent.	Organelles and the cytoskeleton (a network of filaments and filaments) are found.

The nucleus, which is surrounded by a double membrane nuclear envelope, is the biggest cellular organelle. The outer membrane is connected to the endoplasmic reticulum membranes. The two nuclear membranes feature nuclear holes with a diameter of around 90 nm at regular intervals. These holes allow products generated in the nucleus to freely flow into the surrounding cytoplasm.

DNA, the reservoir of genetic information, is found in the nucleus. Nucleosomes are made up of eukaryotic DNA and basic proteins (histones) in a 1:1 ratio. Chromatin fibres of chromosomes are made up of nucleosomes. A single human chromosome thus has around a million nucleosomes. The number of chromosomes in a species is a distinguishing trait. Humans have 46 chromosomes in their nucleus, which are tightly packed.

The nucleolus is a compact mass found in the nucleus of eukaryotic cells.

It contains a lot of RNA, especially ribosomal RNA, which reaches the cytosol via nuclear pores.

Nucleoplasm is the term used to describe the nucleus's ground material. Enzymes like DNA polymerases and RNA polymerases are abundant.

Cell Organelles

Many membrane-bound organelles in eukaryotic cells carry out specialised biological functions which are necessary for overall growth and development of living organism. The following are the main organelles and their functions:

1. **Nucleus:** The nucleus contains more than 95 percent of the DNA. The nucleus is the cell's command center and houses all of the cell's DNA. The complicated architecture of nuclear pore complexes control protein and nucleic acid ribonucleic acids (RNAs) migration through the nuclear envelope. DNA is coiled into a thick mass called chromatin in the nucleus, which is stained darkly with dyes. The nucleolus is a second dense mass joined to the inner nuclear envelope by a thin membrane. DNA polymerases and RNA polymerases are found in the nucleoplasm of the nucleus and are involved in the synthesis of m-RNA and t-RNA.

   The main functions of nucleus are as follows:

   - The nucleus is where DNA replication and RNA transcription take place. Transcription is the primary metabolic activity of the nucleus and is the initial step in the manifestation of genetic information.

- The nucleolus is non membranous and contains enzymes such as RNA polymerase, RNAase, ATPase, and others, but not DNA polymerase. The nucleolus is where ribosomal RNA is made (r-RNA).

- Ribosome subunits are put together in nucleolus.

2. **Mitochondrion**: Mitochondrion is the power house of the cell. There is just one mitochondrion in certain algae, whereas there are half a million in the protozoan Chaos. The number of mitochondria in a mammalian liver cell ranging from 800 to 2500. A typical mammalian mitochondrion measures 0.2 to 0.8 μm in diameter and 0.5 to 1.0 μm in length. Mitochondrion shape changes throughout time. Mitochondria can take on a variety of forms depending on the metabolic state. Two concentric membranes surround the mitochondrion, each with distinct characteristics and biological activities. Phospholipids make up the majority of the outer mitochondrial membrane, which also contains a significant quantity of cholesterol. Porin, a protein found in abundance in the outer membrane, is also present in large quantities. Phospholipids make up the majority of the outer mitochondrial membrane, which also contains a significant quantity of cholesterol. Porin, a protein found in abundance in the outer membrane, is also present in large quantities. It is now well understood that as mitochondria transition from a resting to a respiring state, they undergo significant modifications. The inner membrane does not fold into cristae during respiration; instead, it seems to shrink, leaving a considerably larger intermembrane gap. The intermembrane gap is the area between the outer and inner membranes. Because tiny molecules may pass readily through the outer membrane, the intermembrane space has a similar ionic composition to the cytoplasm. The mitochondrial matrix is the area surrounded by the inner membrane. Matrix composition: The citric acid cycle and fatty acid oxidation enzymes are both found in the matrix. Several strands of circular DNA, ribosomes, and enzymes are also present in the matrix, which are essential for the production of the proteins encoded in the mitochondrial genome. However, the mitochondrion is not genetically self-contained, and the genes encoding the majority of mitochondrial proteins are found in nuclear DNA. The mitochondrion contains several enzymes involved in glucose, fatty acid, and nitrogen metabolism. Electron transport and oxidative phosphorylation enzymes can also be found in various parts of this cell organelle. The mitochondrion is designed to oxidise NADH (reduced NAD) and FAD quickly. H_2 (reduced FAD) is created during the glycolysis, citric acid cycle, and fatty acid oxidation processes. The energy created is captured and stored in the form of ATP for later usage in the body.

3. **Endoplasmic reticulum (ER):** Eukaryotic cells feature a variety of membrane complexes that are connected by organelles. Protein synthesis, transport, modification, storage, and secretion are all carried out by these organelles. The endoplasmic reticulum (ER) extends from the cell membrane, covers the nucleus, surrounds the mitochondria, and seems to link directly to the Golgi apparatus, varying in form, size, and quantity. Cisternae refer to these membranes and the water channels they contain.

   Endoplasmic reticulum (ER) is divided into two types:

   (i) Ergastoplasm, commonly known as rough-surfaced ER.

   They have ribosomes on them. This form of ER combines with the nuclear envelope's outer membrane near the nucleus.

   (ii) Smooth-surfaced ER: Ribosomes are not connected in smooth-surfaced ER.

   Functions: Rough ER is responsible for the generation of membrane lipids and shell proteins. These proteins are injected into the lumen of the cisternae through the ER membrane, where they are changed and transported throughout the cell.

   Smooth ER function: The smooth endoplasmic reticulum is engaged in the process. In the production of lipids, and in the modification and transport of proteins synthesised in the rough ER.

4. **Golgi complexes (also known as the Golgi apparatus):** Dictyosomes is another name for them. The Golgi complex is a unique stack of smooth-surfaced compartments or cisternae found in each eukaryotic cell. The Golgi complexes, which include flattened, fluid-filled golgi sacs, are generally tightly connected with the ER.

   A proximal or cis compartment, a middle compartment, and a distal or trans compartment make up the Golgi complex. Recent data clearly shows that the complex functions as a one-of-a-kind sorting device that accepts freshly produced proteins from the ER that all include signal or transit peptides.

5. **Lysosomes:** Lysosomes are cellular organelles that house a package of enzymes. The name lysosome comes from the Greek word Gree, which means lysis (loosening). De Duve, a Belgian biochemist, was the first to discover and characterise it as a novel organelle in 1955. The average diameter is 0.4 mm (this varies across microsomes and mitochondria). A lipoprotein membrane separates the rest of the body from them. Lysosomes are found in various quantities and varieties in all animal cells except erythrocytes. The lysosomes have a lower pH than the cytoplasm. The optimum pH for lysosomal enzymes is about 5. The enzyme acid phosphatase is utilised to identify this organelle.

6. **Peroxisomes,** also known as microbodies, are microscopic organelles found in eukaryotic cells. The particles have a diameter of around 0.5 mm. These subcellular respiratory organelles lack energy-coupled electron transport mechanisms and are most likely produced by budding from the smooth endoplasmic reticulum (SER).

Functions: They carry out oxidation processes that create hazardous hydrogen peroxide (H_2O_2), which is eliminated by the enzyme catalase. Also, it was recently discovered that liver peroxisomes contain an extremely active -oxidative system that may oxidise long chain fatty acids (C_{16} to C_{18} or $> C_{18}$).

Chapter 2

Carbohydrates

Carbohydrates are the most common energy source. Carbohydrates are made up of the same 2:1 ratio of hydrogen and oxygen atoms as water. Carbohydrates are essential for metabolism because they provide the body with energy. One gram of glucose is oxidized in the biological system to provide 4 calories of energy. The lactating mammary gland contains lactose, the major sugar contained in milk. Carbohydrate degradation products are utilized to produce fatty acids, cholesterol, amino acids, and other chemicals. Inherited damage of certain enzymes in the metabolic pathways of different carbohydrates can lead to disorders such as galactosemia, glycogen storage disorders (GSDs), lactose intolerance, and more. The amount of carbohydrates in living organisms cannot be exceeded. Most animals and plants in nature have both carbohydrate and lipid energy stores; Carbohydrates are usually available quickly, but lipids are a long-term energy source that is used slowly. Proper control of glucose metabolism is essential for survival. Pastoral animals such as cattle, sheep and goats can convert polysaccharides in grass and other foods into proteins, providing them with an important source of protein for humans. Essential carbohydrate drugs such as streptomycin, as well as paper, building blocks, and fabrics, are all made from cellulose in plants.

Carbohydrates are aldehyde or ketone derivatives of high polyhydric alcohol, formed by hydrolysis. Carbohydrates are divided into four categories: monosaccharides, disaccharides, oligosaccharides, and polysaccharides.

Chemical Properties

The presence of functional groups is responsible for the majority of carbohydrates reactions (-CHO and -CO). Some of the reactions are also caused by the presence of alcoholic group present in carbohydrates.

(a) **Oxidation with mild acids:** Only the aldehyde group is oxidised by weak oxidants like HOBr, resulting in monocarboxylic acids. Because ketose sugars do not produce this reaction, it can be used to differentiate between aldoses and ketoses.

$$\text{Glucose} + \text{HOBr} \longrightarrow \text{Gluconic acid} + \text{HBr}$$

(b) Oxidation with metal hydroxides: Sugars are categorized as either reducing or non-reducing. The oxidant (Ag^+ or Cu^{2+}) is decreased when these reagents oxidize sugar, leading in the creation of a silver mirror or the precipitate of cuprous oxide, respectively. These assays are frequently used to discover aldehyde functional groups, and ketoses are classified as reducing sugars due to the ease with which ketoses and aldoses can be interconverted under the basic conditions of this test.

$$\text{Reducing sugar} \;+\; 2\,Cu(OH)_2 \longrightarrow \text{Oxidised sugar} + 2\,Cu^+$$

$$2Cu^+ + 2\,OH^- \longrightarrow 2\,CuOH \longrightarrow 2\,Cu_2O \;+\; H_2O$$
$$\qquad\qquad\qquad\quad \text{yellow} \qquad\qquad \text{red}$$

(c) Reduction with sodium amalgam: It's a nucleophilic addition reaction in which sodium borohydride reduces the C=O group to alcohols. Alditols are the end product of this process. The carbohydrate is converted to primary alcohol if it is an aldehyde, while it creates secondary alcohol if it is a ketose.

(d) Reaction with acetyl chloride or ester formation: Ability to generate sugar esters, such as acetylation with acetyl chloride, indicates the existence of alcohol groups (CH_3COCl). Because of the alcoholic –OH groups, it may react with anhydrides and chlorides of numerous organic and inorganic acids, such as acetic acid, phosphoric acid, sulphuric, and benzoic acids, to generate esters of the corresponding acids.

(e) Reduction with strong mineral acids: Hexose sugars yield 5-hydroxymethylfurfural when reduced with strong mineral acids. Levulinic acid is formed when this chemical is heated further.

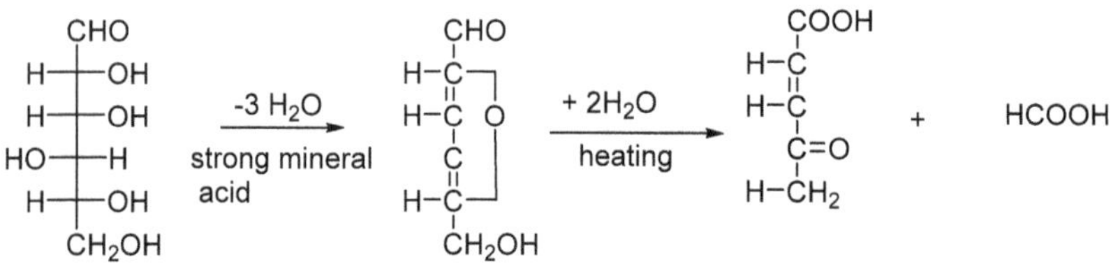

Glucose $\xrightarrow[\text{strong mineral acid}]{-3\,H_2O}$ 5-Hydroxymethyl furfural $\xrightarrow[\text{heating}]{+2\,H_2O}$ Leuvulinic acid $+$ Formic acid (HCOOH)

1. **Monosaccharides** Sugars that cannot be hydrolyzed into a simpler form are referred to be "simple." A typical formula is $C_nH_{2n}O_n$.

    a. Depending on how many carbon atoms they contain, they can be classed as trioses, tetroses, pentoses, hexoses, and so on.

    b. Depending on whether aldehyde (– CHO) or ketone (– CO) groups are present, aldoses or ketoses are formed.

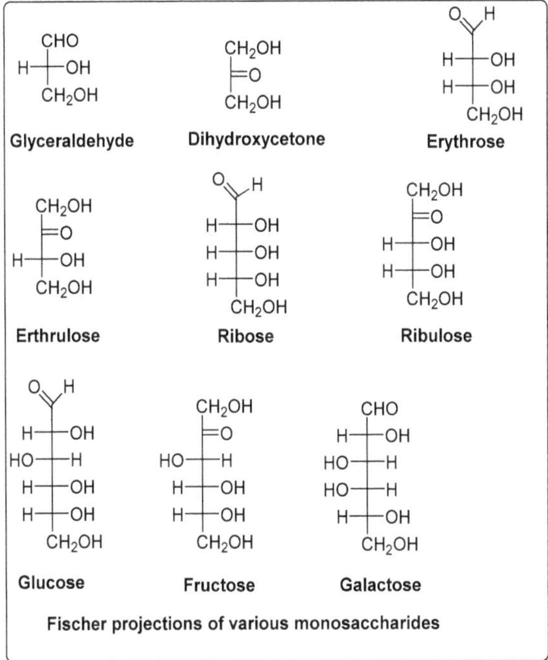

Fig. 2.1 Fischer projections of various monosaccharides.

Glucose: The most prevalent monosaccharide is glucose, which has the molecular formula $C_6H_{12}O_6$. Plants and most algae use sunlight to produce glucose, used to produce cellulose on cell walls, the most common carbohydrate in the biosphere. In all forms of energy metabolism, glucose is the most important energy source. Glucose is stored as a polymer in plants, especially as starch and amylopectin, and in mammals such as glycogen. The glucose circulating in the blood of animals is known as blood sugar.

Fructose, commonly called fruit sugar, is a simple ketonic sugar found in many plants, which is often combined with glucose to form a sucrose disaccharide. It is one of three dietary monosaccharides absorbed directly into the digestive tract after digestion, as well as glucose and galactose. In 1847, French chemist Augustin-Pierre Dubrunfaut discovered fructose. In 1857, an English chemist named William Allen Miller coined the term "fructose." Fructose is a sweet, white, odorless, crystalline substance that is highly soluble in water of all sugars. Fructose is found in honey, fruit and vinegar, flowers, berries, and many root vegetables.

Sugarcane, sugar beet, and corn are all used to extract fructose for commercial purposes. High-fructose corn syrup (HFCS) is a sugar that contains both glucose and fructose. Sucrose is a sugar made up of one glucose molecule and one fructose molecule linked together. Fructose, in all of its forms, including fruits and juices, is frequently used to enhance the palatability and flavor of meals and drinks, as well as to different foods, such as baked goods. About 240,000 tons of crystalline fructose are produced each year.

Eating fructose intake (especially in sugary drinks) has been linked to metabolic syndrome, which includes insulin resistance, obesity, high LDL cholesterol, and triglycerides. According to the European Food Safety Authority, fructose can be substituted for sucrose and glucose in sugary foods and beverages as it has a reduced effect on postprandial blood sugar. "High fructose consumption, on the other hand, may cause metabolic problems such as dyslipidemia, insulin resistance, and increased visceral adiposity," according to the study.

Galactose is a monosaccharide with the chemical formula $C_6H_{12}O_6$, similar to glucose. Apart from the placement of a single hydroxyl group, it has a structure very similar to glucose. Galactose, on the other hand, differs from sugar in its chemical composition and metabolic properties. Galactose is a component that provides energy during time and serves as a necessary basis for the formation of various micromolecules in the body. Galactose is a key component of glycoconjugates, immunological determinants, hormones, cell membrane structures, lectins, and other glycoproteins. Galactose is also involved with galactolipids, which are important components of the central nervous system. Galactose metabolic processes are important not only in the supply of these macromolecules, but also in preventing the accumulation of galactose and galactose metabolites. Galactosemia, or problems with galactose metabolism, can lead to a variety of clinical symptoms in humans.

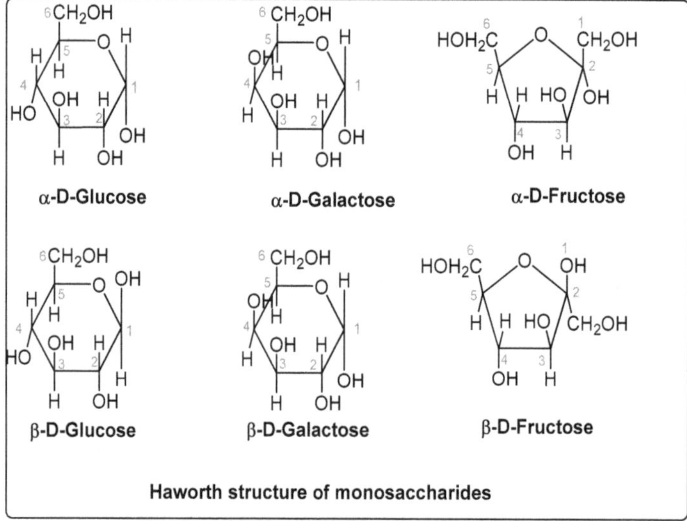

Fig. 2.2 Howarth structures of monosaccharides.

2. **Oligosaccharides** (Greek: oligo-few) are monosaccharide molecules that comprise 2–10 monosaccharide units that are released after hydrolysis. Oligosaccharides are further subdivided into disaccharides, trisaccharides and so on based on the number of monosaccharide units present. In hydrolysis, maltose releases two glucose molecules, while lactose produces one glucose molecule and one galactose molecule.

When sucrose is hydrolysed, it produces one glucose molecule and one fructose molecule.

Reducing and non-reducing sugars:

Reduced sugar is any carbohydrate that can reduce other compounds other than hydrolyzed first, and unsaturated sugars are any sugar that does not have a free ketone or aldehyde group. It is important to note that non-reduced carbohydrates are never oxidized. Sucrose is the most common example of undigested sugar. The most important question you need to answer here is why sucrose is an undigested sugar. The reason for this is that in sucrose, the glycosidic interaction between C-2 carbon fructose and C-1 carbon of glucose binds two units of monosaccharide together very safely. Sucrose is an undigested sugar because the reduced fructose and glucose groups are involved in the formation of glycosidic bonds.

1,2 having chemical formula $C_{12}H_{22}O_{11}$. Sucrose is also known as table sugar and cane sugar. A glycosidic β-(1, 2') link connects the fructose and glucose molecules in a molecule. Glycosidic interaction refers to the fusion of two monosaccharides. Sucrose is a monoclinic crystal structure with high water solubility. It is distinguished by its delicious taste. In 1857, English scientist William Miller coined the term sucrose. It is widely used in food as a sweetener. Because of its delicious taste, refined sucrose (or sugar) is a common part of many food recipes.

Maltose, sometimes referred to as malt, is a disaccharide composed of two glucose units with an α-(1, 4') bond. A glycosidic bond connects the two units of glucose. The enzymes maltase and isomaltase break down maltose molecules into two glucose molecules in the human small intestine mucosa, which are then absorbed by the body. After cellulose, starch is the most abundant carbohydrate in plant cells.

Sucrose, maltose, and lactose are the three most prevalent disaccharides. When one water molecule is removed by connecting two monosaccharides, a disaccharide molecule is created, and the reaction that occurs during this process is called dehydration.

Lactose is a disaccharide formed when galactose and glucose are combined by β-(1,4') glycosidic bond. Lactose is hydrolysed into glucose and galactose, isomerized into lactulose in an alkaline solution, and catalytically hydrogenated into lactitol, a polyhydric alcohol.

Lactulose is a commercially available medication that is used to relieve constipation.

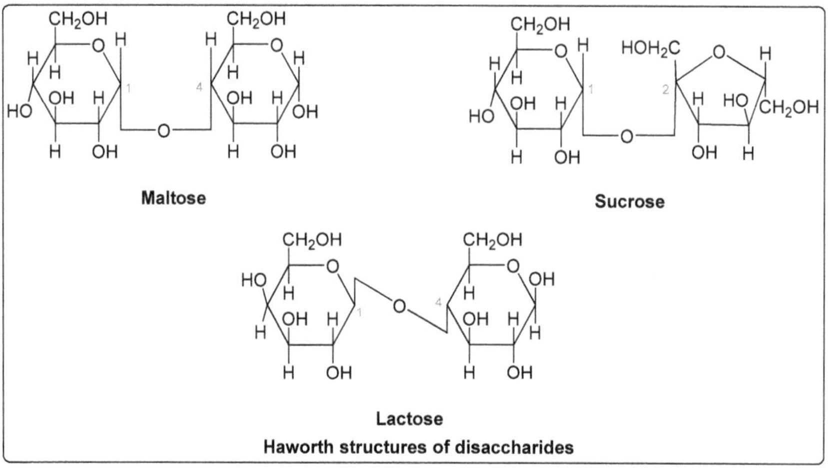

Fig. 2.3 Haworth structures of disaccharides.

3. **Polysaccharides** (Greek: poly-many) are high-molecular-weight polymers of monosaccharide units (up to a million). These are polymerized monosaccharide units made up of multiple monosaccharide units. Polysaccharides aren't sugar carbs since they don't taste sweet. Non-sugars usually have no taste and form colloids when they come into contact with water. Polysaccharides are divided into two categories: homopolysaccharides and heteropolysaccharides.

Homopolysaccharides (homoglycans) are compounds made up of identical monosaccharide units.

Among the examples are starch, glycogen, inulin, cellulose, dextrins, and dextrans.

Heteropolysaccharides (heteroglycans) are polymers composed of different monosaccharide units or derivatives.

Glycosaminoglycans (mucopolysaccharides) are one example.

Polymeric carbohydrate starch, also known as amylum, is made up of many glucose units that are put together by glycosidic bonding. This polysaccharide is produced by many green plants to conserve energy. It is found in large quantities in basic foods such as wheat, potatoes, corn, rice, and cassava, and it is the most common carbohydrate in the human diet worldwide (manioc). Pure starch is a white powder with no odor or taste that does not dissolve in cold water or alcohol. This molecule is made of direct and helical amylose, as well as branching amylopectin.

Glycogen is a more branched version of amylopectin that acts as a storehouse of animal sugar. Starch is converted into sugar, as food, and then fermented to produce ethanol for the production of beer, whiskey, and biofuels. It is used to make a lot of sugar in digested foods. Most starches, such as wheat paste, may be produced into a paste and used as a thickening, stiffening, or glueing agent by mixing them with warm water. The most prevalent non-food use of starch is as an adhesive in the papermaking process. Before ironing, a starch solution can be used to stiffen various materials.

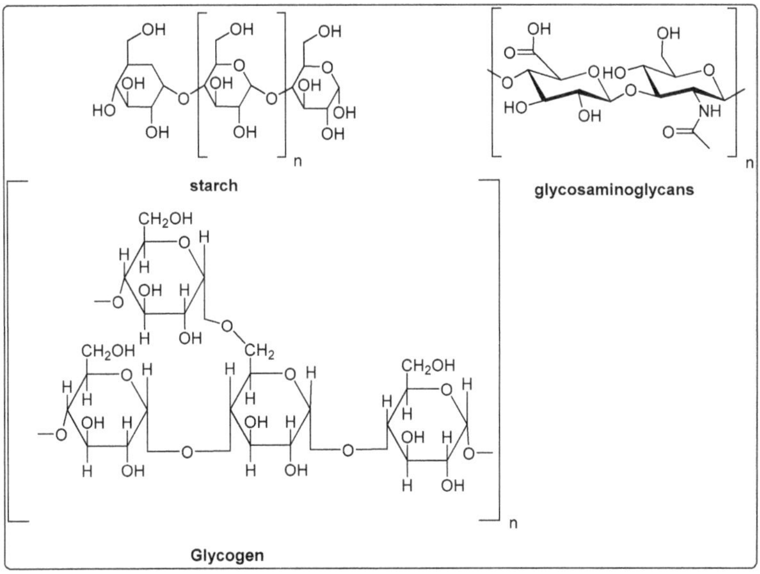

Fig. 2.4 Structures of polysaccharides.

Stereochemistry

Stereoisomers are compounds with the same chemical formula but different spatial arrangements. It is considered asymmetric when a carbon atom is bound to four different atoms or groups. The number of asymmetric carbon (n) atoms, equal to 2n, determines the potential isomers of an object. Because of its four asymmetric carbons, glucose contains 16 isomers.

Glyceraldehyde is a very simple monosaccharide with a single atom of asymmetric carbon (triose). It is present in two stereoisomers and is selected as a reference carbohydrate to indicate the composition of all other carbohydrates.

D and L Isomers

Isomers D and L are very different. The location of the H and OH groups in the carbon atom (C5 glucose) near the terminal primary alcohol carbon determines whether the sugar is D- or L-isomer. If the OH group is on the right, the sugar belongs to series D; if the OH group is on the left side, the sugar belongs to the L series. D- and L-glucose structures based on D- and L-glyceraldehyde, a reference monosaccharide (glycerose). It is worth noting that D-configuration monosaccharides form a large number of monosaccharides that occur naturally in mammal tissues. D-series monosaccharides are converted by cellular enzymes.

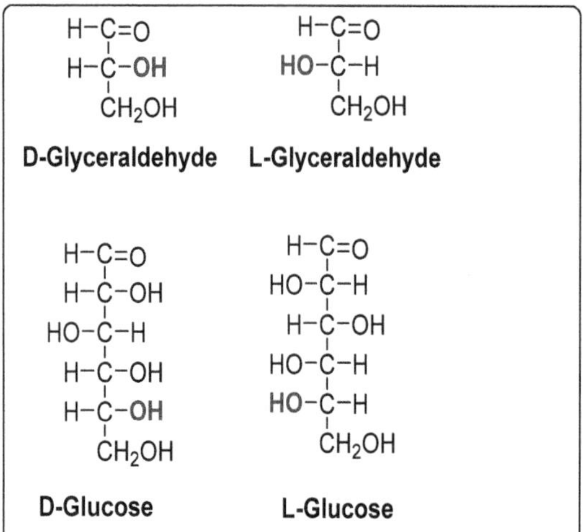

$$
\begin{array}{cc}
\text{H–C=O} & \text{H–C=O} \\
\text{H–C–OH} & \text{HO–C–H} \\
\text{CH}_2\text{OH} & \text{CH}_2\text{OH} \\
\textbf{D-Glyceraldehyde} & \textbf{L-Glyceraldehyde}
\end{array}
$$

$$
\begin{array}{cc}
\text{H–C=O} & \text{H–C=O} \\
\text{H–C–OH} & \text{HO–C–H} \\
\text{HO–C–H} & \text{H–C–OH} \\
\text{H–C–OH} & \text{HO–C–H} \\
\text{H–C–OH} & \text{HO–C–H} \\
\text{CH}_2\text{OH} & \text{CH}_2\text{OH} \\
\textbf{D-Glucose} & \textbf{L-Glucose}
\end{array}
$$

D- and L- forms of glucose compared with D- and L-glyceraldehydes (the reference carbohydrate)

Fig. 2.5 D- and L-forms of glucose.

Qualitative Tests of Carbohydrates

1. **Molisch's test:** This is a test for all carbohydrates in general. **Sulphuric acid** hydrates glycosidic linkages to produce monosaccharides, which are then dehydrated to make furfural and its derivatives in the presence of an acid. Sulphonated-naphthol reacts with these compounds to form a purple complex. Polysaccharides and glycoproteins give a positive reaction as well.

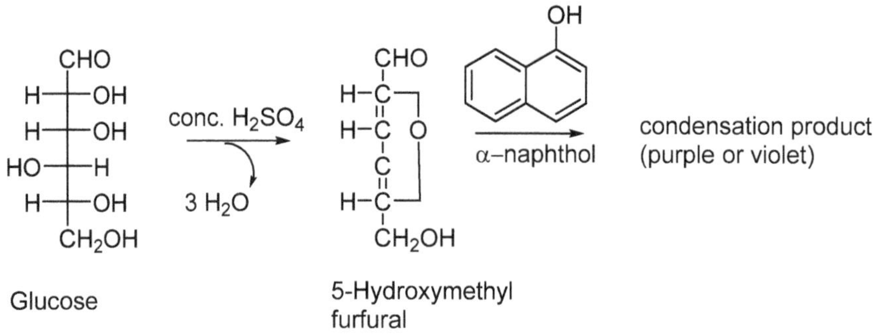

Glucose $\xrightarrow[\text{3 H}_2\text{O}]{\text{conc. H}_2\text{SO}_4}$ 5-Hydroxymethyl furfural $\xrightarrow{\alpha\text{–naphthol}}$ condensation product (purple or violet)

2. **Anthrone test:** Anthrone reaction is another general test for carbohydrates. In this the furfural produced reacts with anthrone to give bluish green coloured complex.

   Procedure: To 2 mL of anthrone reagent, add 0.5-1 mL of the test solution and mix well. Check to see if the color turns to a bluish green. If not, check the tubes once more while immersed in a hot water bath for ten minutes.

Glucose $\xrightarrow[\text{3 H}_2\text{O}]{\text{conc. H}_2\text{SO}_4}$ 5-Hydroxymethyl furfural $\xrightarrow{\text{Anthrone}}$ Bluish-green complex

3. **Iodine test:** With polysacchaides, iodine produces colourful complexes. Iodine turns starch blue, whereas glycogen transforms get changed into a reddish-brown complex. As a result, it is a valuable, practical, and quick test for detecting amylase, amylopectin, and glycogen.

4. **Barfoed's test:** This test is used to clearly differentiate between monosaccharides and reducing disaccharides. Monosaccharides typically react in 1 to 2 minutes, whereas reducing disaccharides take 7 to 12 minutes to hydrolyze and then react with the reagent. This test produces a brick red colour due to the formation of cuprous oxide.

$$(CH_3COO)_2Cu + 2H_2O \longrightarrow 2CH_3COOH + Cu(OH)_2$$

Cupric acetate → Cupric hydroxide

$$Cu(OH)_2 \longrightarrow CuO + H_2O$$

D-Glucose + 2CuO (cupric oxide) $\longrightarrow$ D-Gluconic acid + Cu_2O (Cuprous oxide (red ppt))

5. **Fehling's test:** The Fehling's test is a highly precise and sensitive method for detecting reducing sugars. The presence of reducing sugars is indicated by the formation of yellow or red ppt of cuprous oxide. The chelating agent in this reaction is Rochelle salt.

   Procedure: Add 1mL of Fehling's solution to 1mL of unknown sample. Place the test tubes in a hot water bath after fully mixing. Keep an eye out for the production of a red ppt of cuprous oxide, which indicates that the solution contains reducing sugars.

$$\text{D-Glucose} + 2CuO \longrightarrow \text{D-Gluconic acid} + Cu_2O \text{ (Cuprous oxide, red ppt)}$$

6. **Benedict's test:** Benedict's test (complex mixture of sodium carbonate, sodium citrate and copper sulphate pentahydrate) is easier to use, and this reagent is more stable. Sodium citrate is used as a chelating agent in this method. The presence of reducing carbohydrates causes red ppt of cuprous oxide to develop. To 2 mL Benedict's reagent, add 0.5-1 mL of the test solution or sample extract. In a vigorously boiling water bath, keep the test tubes. Keep an eye out for the production of red precipitates, which could indicate the presence of reducing sugars in the supplied or sample extract.

$$Na_2CO_3 + 2H_2O \longrightarrow 2NaOH + H_2CO_3$$

$$2NaOH + CuSO_4 \longrightarrow Cu(OH)_2 + Na_2SO_4$$

$$Cu(OH)_2 \longrightarrow CuO + H_2O$$

$$\text{D-Glucose} + 2CuO \longrightarrow \text{D-Gluconic acid} + Cu_2O \text{ (Cuprous oxide, red ppt)}$$

Chapter 3

Proteins

In the early nineteenth century, chemists discovered proteins as significant macromolecules, including Swedish scientist Jöns Jacob Berzelius, who coined the term "protein" in 1838, is the Greek word for proteios, meaning "first place." Proteins are specific types, which means they are different from one type to another. Proteins are large, complex molecules that perform various vital functions in the human body. They are essential for the development, function, and regulation of tissues and organs, and are known for spending most of their time in cells. Proteins are made up of thousands or hundreds of tiny components called amino acids that are bound together in long chains. Protein is made up of 20 different amino acids that can be synthesized in a variety of ways. Each protein is a three-dimensional structure and its function is determined by its amino acid sequence. The amino acids are coded by a combination of three building blocks of DNA (nucleotides), which are determined by the sequence of genes.

Biological Significance

Proteins are the primary structural elements of the cytoskeleton. They are the only source of nitrogen replenishment in the body.

- Proteins are biochemical catalysts known as enzymes.
- The transport proteins are in charge of moving substances across membranes and through body fluids.
- Protein is used to make immunoglobulins, which are proteins that serve as the body's first line of defence against bacterial and viral illnesses.
- Structural proteins give mechanical support, whereas contractile proteins like actin and myosin help in the movement of muscle fibres, microvilli, and other structures.
- Proteins that function as receptors can be found in the cell membrane, cytoplasm, and nucleus.
- Storage proteins bind to and store certain chemicals, such as iron (ferritin).
- A few proteins, such as cytochromes, haemoglobin, and myoglobin, are elements of respiratory pigments and are present in the electron transport chain or respiratory chain.

- Proteins may be catabolized to give energy under certain conditions. In addition to the carbon, hydrogen, and oxygen present in carbohydrates and lipids, proteins include nitrogen. Proteins contain roughly 16 percent nitrogen by molecular weight. There's also a little amount of sulphur and phosphorous. A tiny number of proteins include other elements such as I, Cu, Mn, Zn, and Fe. Amino acids are the body's building components. Hydrolysis is a method of dissolving proteins into smaller fragments. Amino acids are the tiny components of proteins known as monomers. Proteins are made up of 20 distinct types of amino acids that are organised in varied patterns and amounts. As a result, nature can and does include an endless number of proteins. As a result, proteins are non-branched L—amino acid polymers.

The L—amino acid has the following general formula:

$$H_2N-\underset{\underset{H}{|}}{\overset{\overset{R}{|}\alpha}{C}}-COOH$$

R is side chain that might be hydrogen, aliphatic, aromatic, or heterocyclic. Each amino acid has an NH_2 amino group, a COOH carboxylic acid group, and a hydrogen atom linked to the carbon close to the – COOH group. As a result, the side chain differs from one amino acid to the next.

Amino Acids: Amino acids are the building blocks of all proteins; these amino acids are held together by peptide bonds (-CONH-), which are responsible for the overarching structure of the protein. In addition to a carboxylic acid group and an amine group, amino acids also include a variable side chain, which varies depending on the kind of amino acid. There are twenty distinct amino acids, all of which have side chains that are distinctive from those of the others. All amino acids, with the exception of glycine, exhibit optical activity due to the presence of an asymmetric carbon atom in their structures. Amino acids arranged in a L– configuration are present in every naturally occurring protein, while amino acids arranged in a D– configuration are found in antibiotics and the cell walls of bacteria. The manner in which amino acids behave in a solution determines their placement in one of three distinct groups.

A. neutral

B. acidic

C. basic

A. Neutral amino acids: This group of amino acids includes aliphatic, aromatic, heterocyclic, and S-containing amino acids. It is the most inclusive of all the categories.

a. Aliphatic amino acids:

Glycine (Gly)	H H–C–COOH NH$_2$	α-amino acetic acid
Alanine (Ala)	H H$_3$C–C–COOH NH$_2$	α-amino propionic acid.
Valine (Val)	H$_3$C C–C–COOH H$_3$C H NH$_2$	α-amino-isovaleric acid.
Leucine (Leu)	H$_3$C H$_2$ H C–C–C–COOH H$_3$C H NH$_2$	α-amino-isocaproic acid.
Isoleucine (Ile)	H$_3$CH$_2$C NH$_2$ C–C–COOH H$_3$C H H	α-amino-β-methyl valeric acid
Serine (Ser)	HO NH$_2$ H$_2$C–C–COOH H	α-amino-β-hydroxy propionic acid
Threonine (Thr)	OHH H$_3$C–C–C–COOH H NH$_2$	α-amino-β-hydroxybutyric acid

b. Aromatic amino acids: Aromatic amino acids make up the second group of neutral amino acids.

Phenylalanine (Phe)	H$_2$H C–COOH NH$_2$	α-amino-β-phenyl propionic acid
Tyrosine (Tyr)	H$_2$H C–COOH NH$_2$	*p*-hydroxy phenylalanine

c. Heterocyclic Amino Acids:

Tryptophan (Trp)	H$_2$H C–COOH NH$_2$	α-amino-β-3-indole propionic acid.
Histidine (His)	O OH NH$_2$	α-amino-β-imidazole propionic acid.

d. Imino Acids:

Proline (Pro)	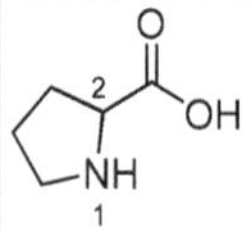	Pyrrolidone-2-carboxylic acid.
Hydroxyproline (Hyp)	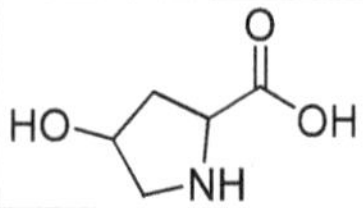	4 hydroxy pyrrolidone-2 carboxylic acid.

e. 'S' containing amino acids: The fourth class includes neutral amino acids containing two sulphur containing amino acids.

Cysteine (Cys)	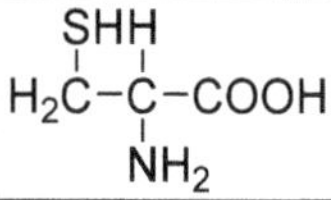	α-amino-β-mercaptopropionic acid
Methionine (Met)	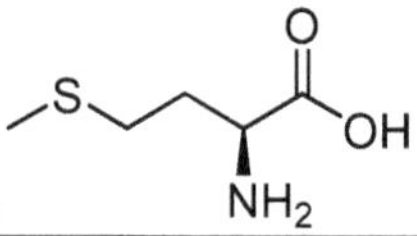	α-amino γ-methylthio-η-butyric acid

B. Acidic amino acids: Amino acids with two –COOH groups and one –NH_2 group are known as acidic amino acids. Therefore, known as monoaminodicarboxylic acids.

Aspartic acid (Asp)	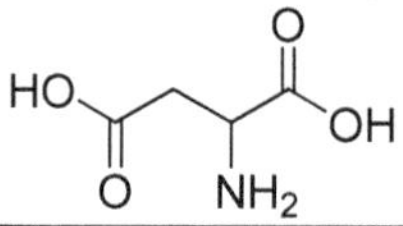	α-amino succinic acid.
Glutamic Acid (Glu)	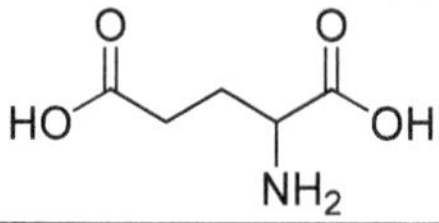	α-aminoglutaric acid

C. Basic amino acids: This category of amino acids includes those with one COOH group and two NH_2 groups. As a result, they're called diamino monocarboxylic acids. This group includes arginine, lysine, and hydroxylysine.

Arginine (Arg)	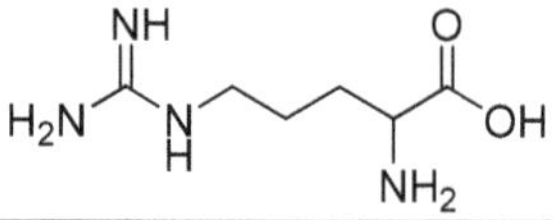	α-amino- δ-guanidino-n-valeric acid
Lysine (Lys)	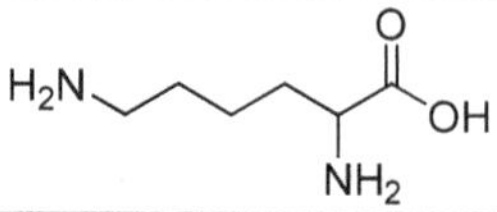	α- ε-diamino caproic acid
Hydroxylysine (Hyl)	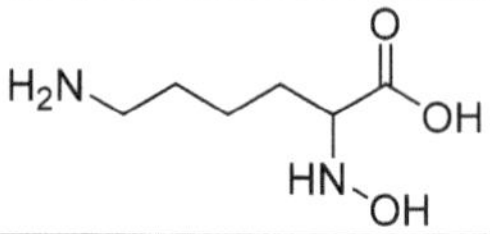	α-ε-diamino-δ-hydroxy-n-valeric acid

Essential Amino Acids

On the basis of nutritional requirement, amino acids are of two types:

- Non-essential amino acids.
- Essential amino acids.
- Semi-essential amino acids.

Essential amino acids are nutrients that cannot be produced by the body and must be absorbed through food. These amino acids include valine, leucine, isoleucine, phenylalanine, threonine, tryptophan, methionine, and lysine.

Non-essential amino acids are those that the body can synthesise, therefore they are not necessary in the diet. Examples of non-essential amino acids are: alanine, arginine, asparagine, aspartic acid, cysteine, glutamic acid, glutamine, glycine, proline, serine and tyrosine.

Semi-essential amino acids: These are growth stimulants because they are not synthesised in appropriate quantities during growth. However, they are essential for developing children, pregnant women, and nursing moms. Arginine and histidine are examples of non-essential amino acids.

The Four Stages of Protein Structural Organisation

Four layers of organisation typically characterise the structure of a protein **(Figure 3.1)**.

Components of Main Significance: A peptide chain's primary structure is made up of a linear succession of amino acids linked together by peptide bonds. These are the most important components. The backbone of a peptide is made up of peptide bonds, whereas the side chains of amino acid residues stick out from the peptide backbone. At the N-terminal end of a terminal amino acid, the -NH_2 group is free, while the -COOH group is free at the C-terminal end. Conventionally, amino acids are numbered starting with 1 from the N-terminal end all the way through to the C-terminal end. In order for a protein to carry out its designated function, it must have a certain set of amino acids in the appropriate proportions. Any change in the sequence is abnormal, and it is possible that this abnormality will have an influence on the protein's function and characteristics.

Secondary Components: By folding or coiling the peptide chain into a three-dimensional secondary structure, the peptide chain can be helical, zigzag, linear, or a combination of these structures. It is caused by the steric interaction between close-proximity amino acids in the peptide chain. Hydrogen bonds and disulfide bonds are the connections or links that contribute to the formation of secondary structures.

Hydrogen bond: Two electronegative atoms, such as O and N, share a single hydrogen atom to create weak, low-energy, noncovalent connections. Secondary structural hydrogen bonds are formed when the oxygen of CO and the nitrogen of -NH of separate peptide bonds share H-atoms. Hydrogen bonding can generate a -helix or a -pleated sheet structure in secondary structure.

- When two cysteine residues join together, disulphide linkages are formed. They are covalent interactions with a great deal of energy and power.

1. **α-Helix**: The alpha-helix is a sequence of regular helical coils that are formed by a peptide chain. These coils are held together by hydrogen interactions between the carbonyl O of the first amino acid and the amide N of the fourth amino acid residues. These interactions are responsible for the stabilisation of the coils. As a direct result of this, there is evidence of intrachain hydrogen bonding in the α-helix. There is the potential for α-helices to be either right-handed or left-handed. Because of steric interference between the C=O and the side chains, the left-handed version of the α-helix is less stable than the right-handed version of the same structure. The right-handed α-helix is the only one that has been found in the structure of proteins. There are 3.6 amino acid residues for every entire turn of the α-helix, and each amino acid residue travels 0.15 nm along the α-helix. The distance of 0.54 nautical miles (nm) that separates two equivalent locations on a turn is referred to as pitch. The alpha helix often contains amino acid residues that are either small or uncharged, such as the amino acids alanine, leucine, and phenylalanine. Polar residues like as arginine, glutamate, and serine have the potential to disrupt the α-helix and make it less stable. Within the alpha-helix itself, proline is never detected. Keratins, a class of α-helical proteins, are present in the proteins of hair, nails, and skin.

2. **β-Pleated Sheet Framework**: Keratins like those that may be found in spider webs, reptile claws, and silk threads make a chain that is almost entirely stretched out. The β-pleated sheet structure conformation is created when hydrogen bonds develop between the carbonyl oxygens and amide hydrogens of two or more continuous extended polypeptide chains. This may occur between two or more polypeptide chains. As a direct consequence of this, hydrogen bonds are able to form between the many chains that make up the β-pleated sheet structure. The structure is not completely flat because of the bond angles; rather, it has a slightly pleated appearance. In the structure of the β-pleated sheet, the adjacent chains may either be parallel or antiparallel. This depends on whether the amino to

carbonyl peptide bonds of the neighbouring chains run in the same direction or the opposite way. The side chains are situated on the opposing sides of the sheet in both the parallel and antiparallel topologies of the β-pleated sheet. The construction of a β-pleated sheet often involves the amino acids glycine, serine, and alanine in the greatest proportions. Proline is present in β-pleated sheets, despite the fact that it has a tendency to make them less stable. by developing kinks Silk fibroin, a kind of protein produced by silkworms, may be found in high concentrations in β-pleated sheets.

3. **Triple helix:** Collagen cannot form α-helix or β-pleated sheet due to its high proline and hydroxyproline content. It generates a helix with three strands. Both noncovalent and covalent interactions contribute to the stability of the triple helix. Interchain hydrogen bonds are formed between peptide chains that are almost perpendicular to the long axis of the α-helix. Additional interchain cross connections and secondary amide bonds of peptide bonds also contribute to the creation of triple helices.

4. **Reverse Turns or β-bends**: Because the polypeptide chain of a globular protein must change direction twice or more when it folds, the conformations that are known as reverse turns or -bends are significant aspects of secondary structure. On the surfaces of globular proteins, where there is minimal steric barrier to prevent the polypeptide chain from reversing orientation, this phenomenon may be seen, reverse turns are most prevalent.

Tertiary structure: A variety of different lengths may be obtained by folding, superfolding, and twisting the polypeptide chain that has the secondary structure that has been described. The term "tertiary structure" refers to this organisational format for a structural plan. There is only one shape that may be considered physiologically active, and proteins in this state are referred to as native proteins. Therefore, the tertiary structure is made up of steric interactions between amino acids that are separated by a significant distance and are brought closer together as a result of folding. Interaction between different groups of amino acids is provided *via* the bonds listed below:

Amino acids that are not polar, such as alanine, leucine, methionine, isoleucine, and phenylalanine, are involved in interactions that are hydrophobic. They are the primary stabilising forces for the tertiary structure, which leads to a compact structure in three dimensions as a consequence of the structure's formation.

- The polar side chains of amino acids are often responsible for the formation of hydrogen bonds.

- Ionic or electrostatic interactions: These are the kinds of interactions that take place between amino acids that have polar side chains that have opposing charges, such acidic and basic amino acids. These are the interactions that take place between side chains that are not polar.
- Disulfide bonds are S–S bonds, which are formed when the -SH groups of two different cysteine residues interact with one another.

In their quaternary structures, a number of different proteins only contain a single chain of peptides. A quaternary structure may be said to exist in a protein if its quaternary structure is composed of two or more peptide chains that are connected to one another by non-covalent interactions or by covalent cross-links. The assembly as a whole is known as an oligomer, whereas each individual peptide chain is known as a monomer or subunit. Oligomeric protein monomers may have similar or distinct primary, secondary, and tertiary structures.

Creatine phosphokinase is a protein consisting of two monomers (dimers) (CPK).

There are two types of proteins that may be classified according to the complexity of their chemical composition: simple and complex.

Amino acids are the building blocks of simple proteins, which are also referred to as homoproteins. Plasma albumin, collagen, and keratin are some examples of substances that fall within this category. Conjugated proteins are sometimes referred to as heteroproteins due to the fact that their structure includes a component that is not a protein. Phosphoproteins, chromoproteins, and glycoproteins are some examples of different types of proteins. Proteins are referred to be glycoproteins when one or more carbohydrate units are covalently linked to the polypeptide backbone of the protein. The branches of plants contain a variety of sugars and carbohydrates, including arabinose, fucose (6-deoxygalactose), galactose, glucose, mannose, N-acetylgluco-samine (GlcNAc, or NAG), and N-acetylneuraminic acid (Neu5Ac or NANA). Glycoproteins include glycophorin, which is the most well-known of the erythrocyte membrane glycoproteins; fibronectin, which binds cells to the extracellular matrix by interacting with collagen or other fibrous proteins on one side and cell membranes on the other; all blood plasma proteins other than albumin; and immunoglobulins or antibodies. Glycoproteins are found in the membranes of erythrocytes.

Proteins that have coloured prosthetic groups added to them are referred to as chromoproteins. Chlorophylls bind a magnesium-centered porphyrin ring, rhodopsins bind retinal, while haemoglobin and myoglobin bind a single heme group and four heme groups, respectively. Rhodopsins bind retinal.

Phosphoproteins are defined as proteins that bind phosphoric acid to residues of serine and threonine. Examples of proteins include dentin, the several caseins found in milk (alpha, beta, gamma, and delta), and phosvitin found in egg yolk. with structural or reserve functions.

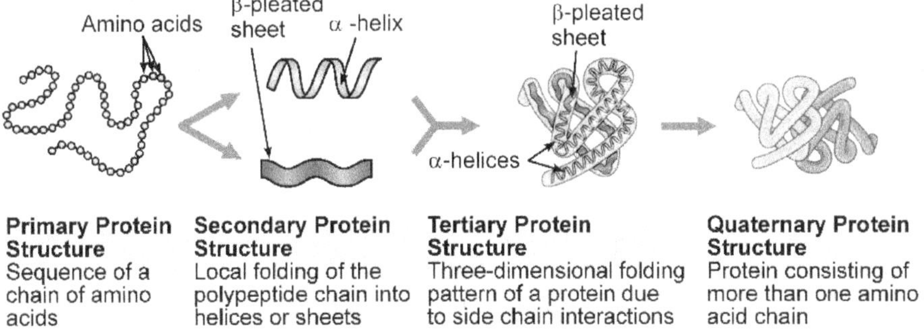

Fig. 3.1 Structure of protein.

Fibrous and globular are the two categories of proteins depending on their form.

Proteins containing a fibrous structure: They sustain both the cells and the entire organism through their primary mechanical and structural functions. These proteins are insoluble in water because they contain an abundance of hydrophobic amino acids both inside and outside. The presence of hydrophobic amino acids on the surfaces of supramolecular structures facilitates their packaging into very intricate structures. In this regard, it is important to note that their polypeptide chains form long filaments or sheets, with one type of secondary structure recurring in the majority of instances. In vertebrates, these proteins offer external protection, support, and form; moreover, their structural characteristics guarantee flexibility and/or strength. Some fibrous proteins, including -keratins, are partly hydrolyzed in the colon. A few examples are shown below.

Spiders and insects create the protein fibroin. This sample is produced by *Bombyx mori*, a silkworm.

Collagen: The term "collagen" refers to a set of structurally related proteins (at least 29 distinct types) that constitute the primary protein component of connective tissue and, more generally, the extracellular framework of multicellular creatures. Approximately 25 to 30 percent of all vertebrate proteins are lipids. They are present in a range of tissues and organs, including tendons and the organic matrix of bone, where they are numerous, as well as cartilage and the cornea of the eye. They produce a variety of structures in various tissues, each of which is able to fulfil an unique need. Molecules in the cornea, for instance, are organised in a nearly crystalline array, rendering it virtually transparent, but in the skin they form fibres that are not highly entangled and directed in all directions, so assuring the skin's tensile strength. Collagen is derived from gelatin, which is utilised in the creation of food.

α-Keratins: They account for almost the whole dry weight of the toenails, claws, beaks, hooves, horns, hair, and wool, as well as a significant percentage of the epidermis that covers the surface of the skin.

The degree to which protein structures are rigid or flexible is directly proportional to the amount of disulfide bonds that, in conjunction with other binding factors, contribute to the stabilisation of the protein structure. Wool keratins are flexible, soft, and extensible in contrast to claw and beak keratins, which have a large number of disulfide connections. This is because wool keratins have a lower number of disulfide links than claw and beak keratins.

Elastin is a protein that contributes to the suppleness of skin as well as blood vessels. The structure of elastin, which is random and coiled, is distinct from that of -keratins and collagens, respectively.

Proteins that are present in the globules include: The vast majority of proteins are classified under this heading. They have a shape that is compact and more or less spherical, and they have a structure that is more complicated than fibrous proteins. Discoveries include not just secondary structures but also motifs, domains, tertiary structures, and even quaternary structures. In general, they are water-soluble; nevertheless, they may also be found integrated into biological membranes (transmembrane proteins), which places them in an environment that is hydrophobic.

Classification on the basis of Solubility and Physical Properties

However, there are many similarities between the two classification categories: On the basis of solubility and physical properties proteins are classified into following categories. As a result, the third most suitable protein classification scheme is used. Proteins are grouped into three types based on their solubility and physical properties, according to this classification scheme.

  A. **Simple proteins**: These are proteins that yield solely amino acids when fully hydrolyzed.

  B. **Conjugated proteins**: These are proteins that have a non-protein component termed a prosthetic group in their structure in addition to amino acids.

  C. **Derived proteins**: These are proteins created by the impact of heat, physical forces, or chemical influences on native proteins.

Qualitative Test of Amino Acids and Proteins

1. **Ninhydrin test:** All α- amino acids react with ninhydrin (triketohydrindene hydrate), a potent oxidising agent, to produce Rhuemann's purple, a purple-coloured product (diketohydrin) in the pH range of 4-8. All primary amines and ammonia react in the same way, but without producing carbon dioxide. Proline and hydroxyproline react with ninhydrin as well, but the result is a yellow-coloured complex rather than a purple one. Other complex structures such as peptides, peptones, and proteins, in addition to amino acids, react positively when reacted with the ninhydrin reaction.

2. **Xanthoproteic acid test:** This test responds to aromatic amino acids including phenyl alanine, tyrosine, and tryptophan. The aromatic phenyl ring is nitrated in the presence of strong nitric acid, yielding yellow coloured nitro-derivatives. The colour changes to orange at alkaline pH due to the ionisation of the phenolic group.

3. **Lead sulphide test:** Amino acids containing sulphur, such as cysteine and cystine on boiling with sodium hydroxide produce sodium sulphide. This reaction occurs as a result of the partial conversion of organic sulphur to inorganic sulphide, which can be observed by precipitating it to lead sulphide in a lead acetate solution.

4. **Hydrolysis:** In the presence of acids, bases, or digestive enzymes, proteins can be partially or totally hydrolyzed. Some or all of the peptide linkages in a protein are broken when it is hydrolyzed. The end products are determined by how long the hydrolysis is allowed to proceed. Peptides are the end products of partial hydrolysis, while amino acids are the end products of complete hydrolysis.

5. **Biuret test:** In a basic solution, compounds having two or more peptide bonds will react with Cu^{2+} to generate a violet-pink complex. Because the original Cu^{2+} solution is blue, the chemical being examined might be either an amino acid or a dipeptide, or neither.

Diseases Related to Malnutrition of Proteins

One of the most serious health issues facing children throughout the globe is an inadequate intake of protein and calories. Protein deficiency may manifest itself in a number of clinical disorders, including kwashiorkor, marasmus, and anaemia.

Kwashiorkor: The protein deficiency illness known as kwashiorkor is characterised by a prolonged period during which an insufficient amount of protein or protein of low quality is consumed. Kwashiorkor causes swelling throughout the body, however it is most noticeable in the face, hands, and feet. Changes may be seen in both the hair and the skin. The hair may grow lighter in colour or get depigmented to a reddish yellow tinge, and it may fall out in some regions. The skin, on the other hand, may exhibit patches, become dry, and peel off.

Marasmus: Marasmus is a disorder that may develop when an individual consumes insufficient amounts of protein and calories in their diet. It is not only a lack of calories that causes kwashiorkor in marasmic children; there are other contributing factors as well. Weight loss and an inability to gain weight are two prominent indicators and symptoms of the disease, as are a reduction in body fat and a loss of muscle mass. In contrast, a kid suffering from kwashiorkor would have a flabby look as well as edoema or swelling throughout the body, but a marasmic infant will have the appearance of being thin and slender. Children who suffer from kwashiorkor and marasmus should consume meals that are rich in both calories and protein, such as milk, rava, porridge, boiled peanuts, dal, and rice. Some of the sources are eggs, guava, soybeans, rice, dal, soybeans, khichri, mixed flour biscuits, sattu, carrot halwa or carrot, sprouted green dal, and sabudana kheer.

Anaemia: A serious problem in terms of health is anaemia, which may be brought on by a deficiency in several nutrients. A deficiency of iron in the diet is the root cause of this condition. The blood loss that occurs during menstruation and the increase in nutritional demands that occurs during pregnancy are two common factors that contribute to anaemia in women and girls. It is essential to consume a diet that is both varied and well-balanced, and one that is abundant in protein, iron, vitamin C, and the B complex. The best sources are green leafy vegetables, drumsticks, green mango, soybeans, rice bran, gingelly seeds, watermelon, and chiku. Dry fruits such as raisins, currants, dates, figs, and prunes are also advised. Eggs are the greatest source of iron and protein, thus anyone who have the financial means to do so should eat eggs regularly.

Chapter 4

Lipids

Lipids are a heterogeneous category of organic compounds found in plant and animal tissues that are related to fatty acids either directly or indirectly. Chemically, they're different forms of esters of various alcohols. Some lipids may contain phosphoric acid, nitrogenous base, and carbohydrates in addition to alcohol and fatty acids. Properties of lipids are as follows:

1. They are water insoluble.
2. Solubility in one or more organic solvents, such as ether, chloroform, benzene, acetone, and others, referred to as fat solvents.
3. Some actual or possible relationship with fatty acids as esters.
4. Possibility of live organisms using it.
5. Lipids are made up of fats, oils, waxes, other similar substances. At room temperature, an oil is a lipid that is liquid. The difference between fats and oils is solely physical. Chemically, they're all glycerol esters with more fatty acids.

Functions of Lipids

Lipids are an important dietary component that serve as a source of energy for the body. Lipid is preferable than carbohydrates as a raw material for combustion in several ways, as it delivers more energy per gramme (9.5 C/gm vs. 4.0 C/gm for carbohydrates).

1. Unlike carbohydrates, it may be stored in nearly limitless amounts in the body.
2. Lipid deposits in the body may act as an insulator, while lipids around internal organs such as the kidney, for example, may offer padding and protect the organs.
3. Materials for construction: Fat breakdown products can be used to create biologically active materials.
4. Lipids provide so-called essential fatty acids (EFA), which cannot be synthesised by the body and are required for good health and growth in the diet.

5. Lipids are abundant in the neurological system, especially certain kinds, and are required for normal function.

6. Because several vitamins, such as A, D, E, and K, are fat soluble, lipid is required for their absorption.

7. Lipoproteins and phospholipids are significant components of a variety of natural membranes, including cell walls and cell organelles such as mitochondrion.

8. Triglycerides, cholesterol, and PL are all carried by lipoproteins in the body.

Classification of Lipids

They can be classified based on their physical qualities at room temperature (solid or liquid, respectively for fats and oils), their polarity, or their human requirement, although the structure is the preferable criterion.

On the basis of their structure, they may be categorised into three groups.

Simple lipids: In its finest form, this category of lipids has two different structural moieties. Esters of long-chain fatty acids and long-chain alcohols, such as triacylglycerols and mono- and diacylglycerols; cholesteryl esters, which are esters of cholesterol and fatty acids; and waxes, which are esters of long-chain fatty acids and fatty acids, such as esters of vitamins A and D.

Complex lipids: There are more than two unique kinds of structural moieties present in complex lipids. They consist of phospholipids, which are glycerol esters of fatty acids, phosphoric acid, and other nitrogen-containing groups; phosphatidic acid, which is diacylglycerol esterified to phosphoric acid; phosphatidylcholine, which is phosphatidic acid connected to choline; and lecithin, phosphatidylethanolamine, phosphatidylserine, and phosphatidyl.

Derived lipids: They either exist as such or are freed from the other two main groups by the process of hydrolysis. Lipids, both simple and complex, are constructed from these building blocks. Included in this category are hydrocarbons, sterols, fatty acids and alcohols, as well as the fat-soluble vitamins A, D, E, and K.

Tri-glycerides: These are the most widespread and typical lipids. These are occasionally referred to as basic fats or oils. These are the primary constituents of the fats that the body stores. These are prevalent in the body's fatty tissues. Tri-glycerides are glycerol esters containing three molecules of fatty acid. Triglycerides are a form of energy storage in the human body.

$$
\begin{array}{lllll}
CH_2OH & + & HOOCR & & CH_2OOCR \\
| & & & -3H_2O & | \\
CHOH & + & HOOCR' & \longrightarrow & CHOOCR' \\
| & & & & | \\
CH_2OH & + & HOOCR'' & & CH_2OOCR'' \\
\end{array}
$$

Glycerol   Fatty acids   Triacyl-glycerol (or triglyceride)

Triglycerides are virtually nonpolar molecules that have long carbon chains and do not dissolve easily in polar solvents such as water. Triglycerides also have a high melting point. On the other hand, oils and fats are soluble in nonpolar organic solvents such as hexane and ethers. These solvents include: Triglycerides are the primary source of energy that is stored in animals. They originate in the foods that we consume, namely butter, oils, and other types of fats. The primary cause of elevated triglyceride levels is also the consumption of more calories. These are calories that a person takes into their body, but that their body does not immediately need. If all three of the hydroxyl groups on the glycerol molecule are esterified with the same kind of fatty acid, such as tripalmitin, then the lipid in question is referred to as simple triacyl glycerol. Mixed glycerides, such as dioleopalmitin, are formed through esterification of various fatty acids.

Triglyceride levels can be raised by a variety of factors, including:

- Being overweight or obese
- Cigarette smoking
- Excessive alcohol usage
- Certain drugs
- Thyroid illnesses
- Type 2 diabetes with poor management
- Genetic disorders
- Diseases of the liver or kidneys

A blood test is commonly used to evaluate triglycerides and cholesterol in the body. Milligrams per deciliter (mg/dL) is the unit of measurement for triglycerides. The following are triglyceride guidelines:

- Less than 150 milligrammes per deciliter (mg/dL) or 1.7 millimoles per litre (mmol/L) is considered normal.
- 150 to 199 mg/dL (1.8 to 2.2 mmol/L) is considered borderline high.

- High (2.3–5.6 mmol/L) — 200–499 mg/dL
- 500 mg/dL or more (5.7 mmol/L or more) is considered extremely high.

Physical Properties of Triglycerides

- They are non-polar, hydrophobic, water insoluble, and organic solvent soluble.
- The specific gravity is lower than that of water. Fats and oils float on water as a result.
- They act as a solvent for other fats. Vitamins A, D, E, and K, for example, are fat-soluble vitamins.
- Saturated fatty acids melt at a higher temperature than unsaturated fatty acids of the same length.

Fatty Acids

Within the body, fatty acids have several purposes, one of which is the storage of energy. Fatty acids are converted into energy by the body at times when glucose, another kind of sugar, is in insufficient supply. The lipids of plants, animals, and microbes all include an essential component called fatty acid (fat-soluble components of living cells). In general, a fatty acid is made up of a linear chain that has an even number of carbon atoms, hydrogen atoms that run the length of the chain, and a carboxyl group (COOH) that is located at the other end of the chain. Because it has a carboxyl group, it has the characteristics of an acid (carboxylic acid).

Saturated and unsaturated fatty acids are as follows:

In saturated fatty acid, every carbon-to-carbon link is a single bond. The saturated fatty acids with 16 and 18 carbons, generally known as palmitic acid and stearic acid, are the most extensively distributed. Palmitic and stearic acids are components of the lipids found in the vast majority of organisms. Palmitic acid accounts for up to 30 percent of the total amount of fat found in mammalian bodies. It makes up anywhere from 5 to 50 percent of the lipids found in vegetable fats, although it is found in particularly high concentrations in palm oil. Stearic acid is found in high concentrations in a wide range of vegetable oils (such cocoa butter and shea butter, for example), and it makes up a sizeable component of the lipids in ruminant tallow.

Table 4.1 Some important saturated fatty acids.

Common name	IUPAC name	Number of carbon atoms	Structure
Butyric acid	n-Butanoic acid	4	
Valeric acid	n-Pentanoic acid	5	
Caproic acid	n-Hexanoic acid	6	
Caprylic acid	n-Octanoic acid	8	
Palmitic acid	n-Hexadecanoic acid	16	
Stearic acid	n-Octadecanoic acid	18	

Unsaturated fatty acids are characterised by the presence of one or more double or triple bonds within the acid, which contributes to the reactive nature of the fatty acids. Some fatty acids have branched chains, while others have ring structures. Fatty acids may be divided into three categories: (e.g., prostaglandins). Triglycerides are the most common form in which fatty acids are found in nature. Triglycerides are a combination of fatty acids and glycerol. Free-floating fatty acids are not found in nature. Triglycerides are (an alcohol). The C=C double bonds are responsible for the generation of the cis and trans isomers. In a cis form, the two hydrogen atoms that are next to the double bond project outward from the same side of the chain as the double bond. The double bond's stiffness freezes its shape and, in the case of the cis isomer, forces the chain to bend, limiting the fatty acid's conformational freedom (**Figure 4.1**). The adjacent two hydrogen atoms in a trans configuration, on the other hand, are on different sides of the chain. As a result, they don't bend the chain as much as straight saturated fatty acids do, and their form is similar to that of straight saturated fatty acids.

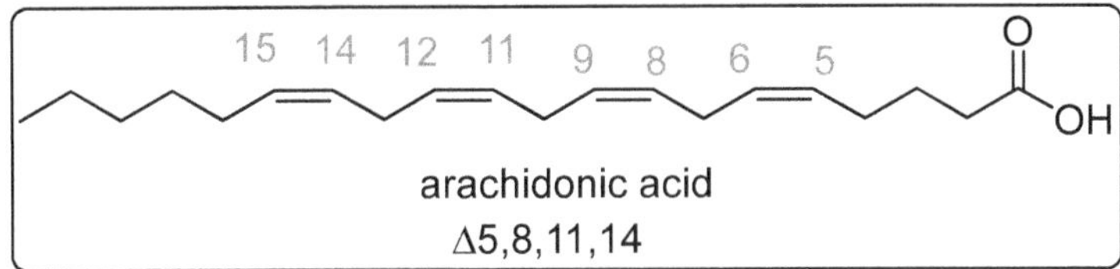

Fig. 4.1 Cis and trans configuration.

A fatty acid having double bonds at locations x,y,.... is conventionally denoted by the notation x,y,.... (The Greek character "Δ" (delta) corresponds to the Roman letter "D," which stands for "double bond.") For example, the 20-carbon arachidonic acid is Δ5,8,11,14 indicating that it has double bonds between carbons 5 and 6, 8 and 9, 11 and 12, and 14 and 15 (**Figure 4.2**).

Fig. 4.2 Naming of Arachidonic acid.

Table 4.2 Important unsaturated fatty acids

Common name	Category	Carbon number	Double bond positions
Palmitoleic acid	Monoenoic acid	16	9;10
Oleic acid		18	9;10
Elaidic acid		18	9;10
Nervonic acid		24	15;16
Linoleic acid	Dienoic acid	18	9;10, 12;13
Archidonic acid	Tetraenoic acid	20	5;6, 8;9, 11;12, 14;15

Essential Fatty Acids

Essential fatty acids, also known as EFA, are a kind of polyunsaturated fatty acid known as PUFA. The body is unable to synthesise essential fatty acids, but they are necessary for maintaining good health and must be received from food. There are two categories of EFAs: omega-3 (also written as -3) and omega-6 (also written as -6). In omega-3 fatty acids, the last carbon–carbon double bond is located in the -3 position, which indicates that it is the third bond from the methyl end of the fatty acid. On the other hand, in omega-6 fatty acids, the last carbon–carbon double bond is located in the -6 position, which indicates that it is the sixth bond from the methyl end of the fatty acid. Essential fatty acids, sometimes referred to as EFAs, are a kind of fatty acid that cannot be produced by the bodies of humans or other animals, hence these acids must be consumed instead. Fatty acids that are required for various biological processes are referred to as essential fatty acids. This distinction is made in contrast to fats that serve primarily as sources of energy in the body. Essential fatty acids are not to be confused with essential oils, which are considered "essential" because they contain a highly concentrated form of the essence of the plant or flower they come from. Only two types of fatty acids are necessary for humans: alpha-linolenic acid, which is an omega-3 fatty acid, and linoleic acid, which is an omega-6 fatty acid (an omega-6 fatty acid). Other fatty acids, such as docosahexaenoic acid, which is an omega-3 fatty acid, and gamma-linolenic acid are sometimes categorised as "conditionally essential," which means that they can become necessary under certain conditions, such as during certain stages of development or when an individual is ill (an omega-6 fatty acid). When they were first discovered in 1923, the two EFAs were given the name "vitamin F." However, research conducted on rats in 1929 demonstrated that they are more appropriately classified as fats rather than vitamins.

Cholesterol

The production of steroid hormones, vitamin D, and bile acids all need cholesterol as an essential ingredient. Cell membranes include cholesterol, which functions as a structural component. Cholesterol has an essential function in the regulation of cellular activity in addition to the structural role it plays in the maintenance of fluidity and stability. Cholesterol is a molecule that is composed of 27 carbons and has a hydrocarbon tail, a sterol nucleus that is comprised of four hydrocarbon rings, and a hydroxyl group. Steroid hormones are characterised by the presence of a sterol nucleus or ring at the core of their structure. Due to the fact that they are non-polar, the hydrocarbon tail and the core ring do not dissolve in water. As a direct consequence of this, cholesterol, which is a lipid, becomes attached to apoproteins, which are proteins, and is then transported through the circulation as a lipoprotein. Cholesterol makes up more than thirty percent of the material that makes up the membranes of all animal cells. It is necessary for the creation of membranes, their preservation, and the control of fluidity over the whole temperature spectrum of the physiological environment. The hydroxyl group of each molecule of cholesterol and the polar heads of each phospholipid and sphingolipid in the membrane are both responsible for interacting with the water molecules that surround the membrane. Within the membrane are entangled not only the cumbersome steroid and hydrocarbon chains, but also the nonpolar fatty-acid chains of the other lipids. By interacting with phospholipid fatty-acid chains, cholesterol improves membrane packing, which in turn reduces membrane fluidity while maintaining membrane integrity. As a result, animal cells do not need the production of cell walls (like plants and most bacteria). Animal cells are able to adapt their form and animals are able to move as a direct result of the membrane's ability to be tough without being stiff. Cholesterol makes up more than thirty percent of the material that makes up the membranes of all animal cells. It is necessary for the creation of membranes, their preservation, and the control of fluidity over the whole temperature spectrum of the physiological environment. The hydroxyl group of each molecule of cholesterol and the polar heads of each phospholipid and sphingolipid in the membrane are both responsible for interacting with the water molecules that surround the membrane. The thick steroid and hydrocarbon chain, in addition to the other lipids' nonpolar fatty-acid chains, are embedded deep into the membrane.

Lipoproteins

Complex lipids known as lipoproteins are made up of cholesteryl ester and triacylglycerol and are encased in a single molecule of amphipathic phospholipid and cholesterol. They are unique in that they are amphipathic, meaning that they have ends that are polar as well as ends that are non-polar. These biomolecules are made up of lipid and protein molecules, and they are the ones that make it possible for fat molecules to pass through water molecules both within and outside of cells.

All of the phospholipid molecules in a lipoprotein have their polar ends facing outward in order to interact with water, which is also a polar molecule. This enables the lipoprotein to be carried into the circulation, as opposed to rising to the top of the milk like cream. Despite being insoluble in blood, the non-polar fat coiled inside the phospholipid layer at the centre of the lipoprotein is transported by the circulation to the location where it must be stored or processed. Therefore, lipoproteins are molecular transporters that carry fats to locations where they are required or stored. Based on apolipoproteins, which are proteins attached to the phospholipid outer layer, lipoproteins are differentiated. This stabilises the fatty molecule and, in some circumstances, binds to cell surface receptors, allowing the cell to take up the lipoprotein via receptor-mediated endocytosis.

On the basis of their density and the ratio of protein to lipid molecules, lipoproteins are divided into four groups. Lipids exist in several forms, including:

LDL is low-density lipoprotein, a subtype of cholesterol. It is also referred to as "bad cholesterol." A LDL cholesterol level of 100 mg/dL or less is optimal for the majority of individuals. Plaque builds up in the blood vessels as LDL levels rise, which might lead to further cardiac issues.

HDL High-density lipoprotein, sometimes known as good cholesterol, has a high ratio of lipids to proteins. It works by preventing cholesterol accumulation in the arteries. HDL cholesterol levels more than 60 mg/dL are considered optimal.

VLDL are a subtype of very low-density lipoproteins. These lipoproteins are produced by the liver for the export of triacylglycerols.

IDLs is intermediate density lipoprotein is another category of a lipoprotein. These lipoproteins result from the breakdown of VLDL (very-low-density lipoproteins).

Qualitative Tests for Lipids

1. **Solubility test:** Separately add the following organic solvents to tiny amounts of fat/fatty acid in a separate test tube: (3 mL/ test tube) chloroform, ether, benzene, and hexane. If the sample gets completely soluble in the four solvents, it indicates whether or not the provided solution contains fat or oil.

2. **Translucent Spot Test:** The translucent spot test, which is characterised by a translucent and oily spot, is also a preliminary lipids test. Unlike water, the lipid will not moisten the filter paper. Because of their greasy nature, the lipids will permeate the filter paper and produce a greasy or transparent spot. Unlike lipids, the water stain on the paper will vanish.

3. **Saponification Test:** In the presence of ethanol, fatty triglycerides react with an alkali NaOH to form soap and glycerol. Alkaline esters hydrolysis is another name for this process. In this method, test tube is halfway filled with lipid, followed by heating on water bath for 5 minutes in the presence of sodium hydroxide. Finally, ethanol should be added. If froth forms in the test tube, the reuslt indicates presence of lipid in the sample.

4. **Sudan IV test:** The Sudan IV test is used to determine whether or not a solution contains lipid. The notion of lipid binding and solubility in

non-polar substances underpins this test. Sudan IV is a non-polar stain, therefore the lipid will attach to it and keep the colour, resulting in a red-orange stain. Sudan IV is non-staining and non-binding to polar molecules. In this method, test tube is filled with lipid sample, followed by addition of 1-2 drops of Sudan IV to the solution. Appearance of reddish-orange colour in the test-tube confirms the presence of lipid.

5. **Acrolein test:** The acrolein test is used to check for presence of lipid in the unknown sample. The dehydration process, in which water molecules are eliminated from glycerol by adding the reagent potassium hydrogen sulphate, provides the basis for this test. The reaction of glycerol with potassium hydrogen sulphate produces acrolein, which is distinguished physically by the production of a strong odour. In this method, test tube is filled with 1 mL of the lipid sample, followed by addition of potassium hydrogen sulphate and heating of the solution. Strong pungent smell confirms the presence of lipid in the sample.

Chapter 5

Nucleic Acids

Nucleic acids may be defined as long chain polymers of nucleotides or polynucleotides which are bound together by 3' and 5' phosphate links. The major nucleic acids are DNA (deoxyribonucleic acid) and RNA (ribonucleic acid).

Functions of Nucleic Acids

- The main role of nucleic acids is to inherit and transmit individual genetic characters from one generation to the other.

- They also serve as repositories of genetic information.

- DNA controls the many features of cellular functions. DNA is arranged into genes which are known as fundamental structural and functional unit of genetic information.

- Nucleic acids experience mutations.

- Protein synthesis is controlled by genes through the conciliation of RNA as displayed below:

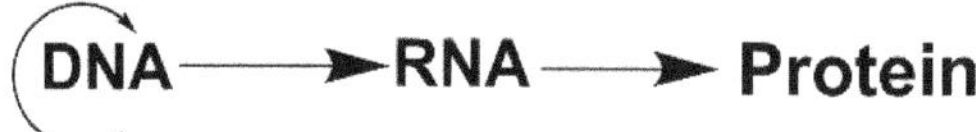

Fig. 5.1 Figure showing central dogma of life process.

- The interrelationship between DNA, RNA and protein forms the central dogma of life or central dogma of molecular biology **Fig. 5.1**.

Purine and Pyrimidine Bases

Nitrogenous bases present in nucleotides or nucleic acids are generally aromatic heterocyclic compounds and are of two types—purines and pyrimidines. The pyrimidines are numbered in the clockwise direction whereas purines are numbered in the anticlockwise direction. Although 5th carbon atom is similar in both bases. The basic nucleus and numbering pattern of pyrimidine and purine bases is shown in **Fig. 5.2**.

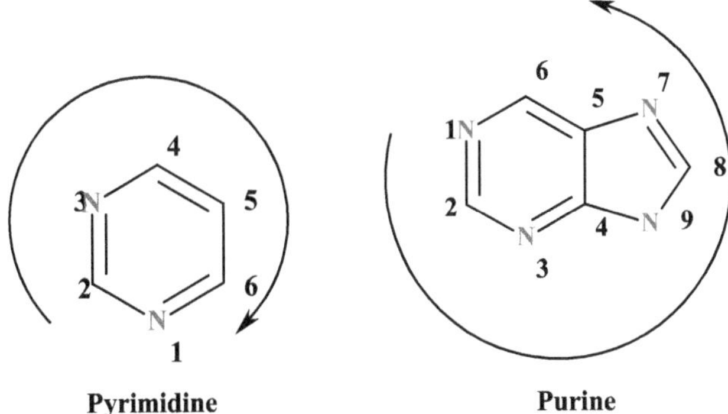

Pyrimidine   **Purine**

Fig. 5.2 Figure showing basic nucleus and numbering pattern of pyrimidine and purine bases.

Components of Nucleosides and Nucleotides

Nucleotides consist of a nitrogenous base, a pentose sugar moiety and a phosphate group. Nucleosides consist of a base and a sugar moiety. Therefore, nucleotide can be referred to as nucleoside + phosphate group.

Nucleoside = Nitrogenous Base + Sugar Moiety

Nucleoside = Nucleotide – Phosphate group

Nucleotide = Nucleoside + Phosphate group

Nitrogenous Bases

The major purine bases consist of adenine (A) (6-aminopurine) and guanine (G) (2-amino-6-oxypurine) whereas pyrimidine bases are composed of cytosine (C) (2-oxy-4-aminopyrimidine), thymine (T) (2,4-dioxy-5-methylpyrimidine) and uracil (U) (2,4, -dioxypyrimidine). The chemical structures of nitrogenous bases are shown in **Fig. 5.3**.

Adenine (A)   **Guanine (G)**

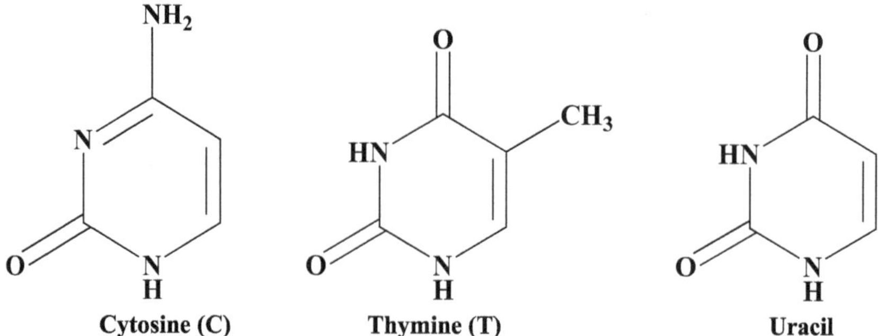

Fig. 5.3 Chemical structures of nitrogenous bases (purines and pyrimidines).

Sugars Moiety

The nucleic acid structure contains pentoses or five carbon monosaccharides (pentoses). RNA is composed of D-ribose whereas DNA contains D-deoxyribose. Both the sugars i.e., ribose and deoxyribose vary in their structure at C2 position. Deoxyribose has one oxygen less at C2 compared to ribose. The chemical structures of ribose and deoxyribose sugars are shown in **Fig. 5.4**.

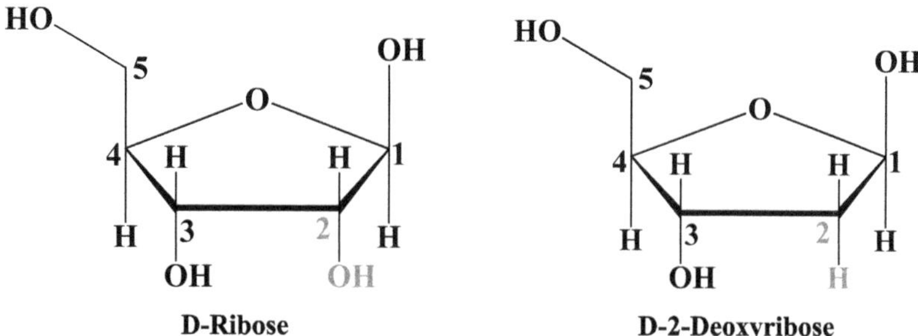

Fig. 5.4 Chemical Structures of ribose and deoxyribose sugars.

Phosphate Group

The phosphate group (PO$_4$) attached to C5 position of sugar moiety differentiates nucleoside from nucleotide. These phosphate groups form phosphodiester bonds with the pentose sugars to build up the sides of the DNA "ladder".

Nomenclature of Nucleosides and Nucleotides

When pentose sugar is added to a base it produces a nucleoside. Ribonucleosides are produced, when the sugar is ribose. Ribonucleosides of A, G, C and U are called as adenosine, guanosine, cytidine and uridine respectively.

Deoxyribonucleosides are formed when the sugar is deoxyribose. The term mononucleotide is used when a single or multiple phosphate moiety is attached to a nucleoside i.e., known as mononucleotide. Simplest example is adenosine monophosphate (AMP) which contains an adenine base, a ribose sugar and a phosphate group. The chemical structures of nucleoside (adenosine) and nucleotide (AMP) are shown in **Fig. 5.5.**

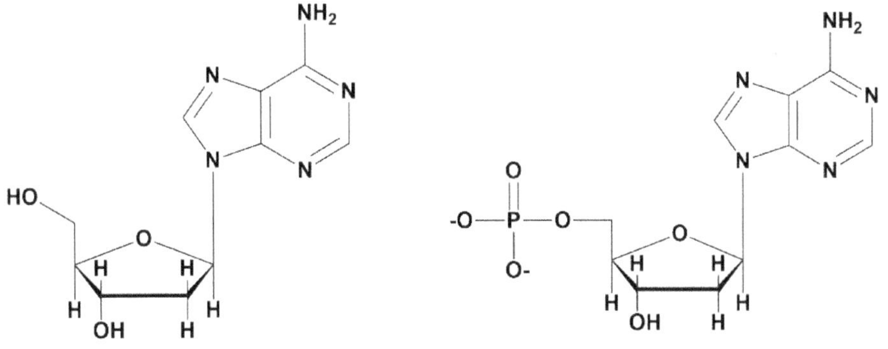

Adenosine
(Nucleoside)

Adenosine Monophosphate (AMP)
Nucleotide)

Fig. 5.5 Chemical structures of nucleoside (adenosine) and nucleotide (AMP).

Structure of DNA (Watson and Crick Model)

Swiss biologist Johannes Friedrich Miescher discovered DNA in during his research on white blood cells in the year 1869. Later in 1953, James Watson and Francis Crick elucidated right-handed double stranded helical structure of DNA **(Fig. 5.6)**. The salient features of double helix DNA model described by Watson and Crick are given below:

- It contains two polydeoxyribonucleotide strands or chains which are curled around each other on common pivot.

- These two strands are joined together by hydrogen bonds.

- The nucleotides bases are paired complementary to each other as adenine(A) to thiamine (T) whereas guanine (G) is paired with cytosine (C).

- A biochemist named Erwin Chargaff found that bases are present in equal amount in DNA double helix.

- According to Chargaff's rule adenine amount present is equal to that of thiamine whereas guanine amount is equal to cytosine ($A=T$ and $G \equiv C$). That means they should be present in the ratio of 1:1.

- The two strands of DNA are antiparallel to each other i.e., one strand moves in 5' to 3' direction whereas other strand moves in 3' to 5' direction.

- The diameter or width of DNA double helix is 2nm (20Å). Ten base pairs of nucleotides are accommodated in each turn of the double helix having length 3.4nm (34Å).

- The genetic information is present in one strand which is called as template strand and the other strand is treated as coding strand which is similar to RNA transcript and encodes the protein.

- There are six conformations of DNA double helix i.e., from A-E and Z.

- The DNA double helix modes elucidated by Watson and Crick is of B-form.

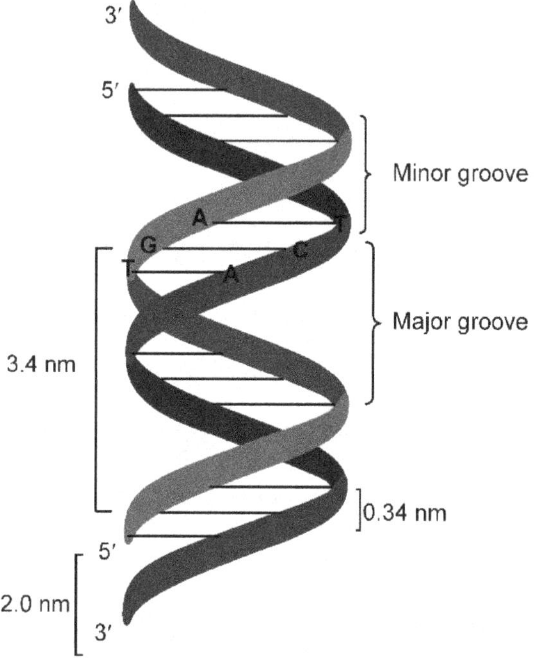

Fig. 5.6 Watson and Crick model of DNA double helix

Functions of DNA

- It carries genes of hereditary information from one generation to another.

- It helps in replication process which is essential for transferring genetic information.

- It undergoes mutation and recombination process.

- DNA undergoes gene expression through which gene encodes genetic information.

Structure of RNA

RNA is the genetic material of majority of viruses and organisms. Its structure is composed of nucleotides i.e., base, ribose sugar attached to phosphate group. The nitrogenous bases present in RNA are adenine, uracil, cytosine and guanine. The thiamine present in DNA is replaced by uracil in RNA. The three main classes of RNA which exist in prokaryotic and eukaryotic organisms are:

1. **Messenger RNA (mRNA)** - It is formed in eukaryotic nucleus as heterogenous nuclear RNA or hRNA. The clarification of hRNA gives rise to mRNA which moves to cytoplasm for contribution in protein synthesis process. The major biological role of mRNA is the synthesis of proteins by transferring genetic information from genes to ribosomes.

2. **Transfer RNA (tRNA)** – The key function of tRNA is to shift amino acids to mRNA for the synthesis of mRNA. The structure of tRNA appears like clover leaf.

3. **Ribosomal RNA (rRNA)** – rRNA is responsible for the contribution of structural framework for ribosomes which help in protein synthesis process. They are also believed to be help in attaching mRNA to ribosomes.

The difference between DNA and RNA is discussed in **Table 5.1** and pictorially represented in **Fig. 5.7**.

Table 5.1 Difference between DNA and RNA

Sr. No.	DNA	RNA
1	Sugar present in DNA is deoxyribose therefore it is known as deoxyribonucleic acid.	Sugar present in RNA is ribose so it is known as ribonucleic acid.
2	It is double-stranded molecule.	It is single-stranded molecule.
3	It replicates itself.	It is synthesized from DNA.
4	It contains base pairs as adenine, thymine, cytosine and guanine.	Thymine is replaced by uracil.
5	It is stable under basic conditions.	It is not stable under alkaline conditions.
6	The main function of DNA is to store and transfer genetic information.	It helps in protein synthesis and codes for amino acids.

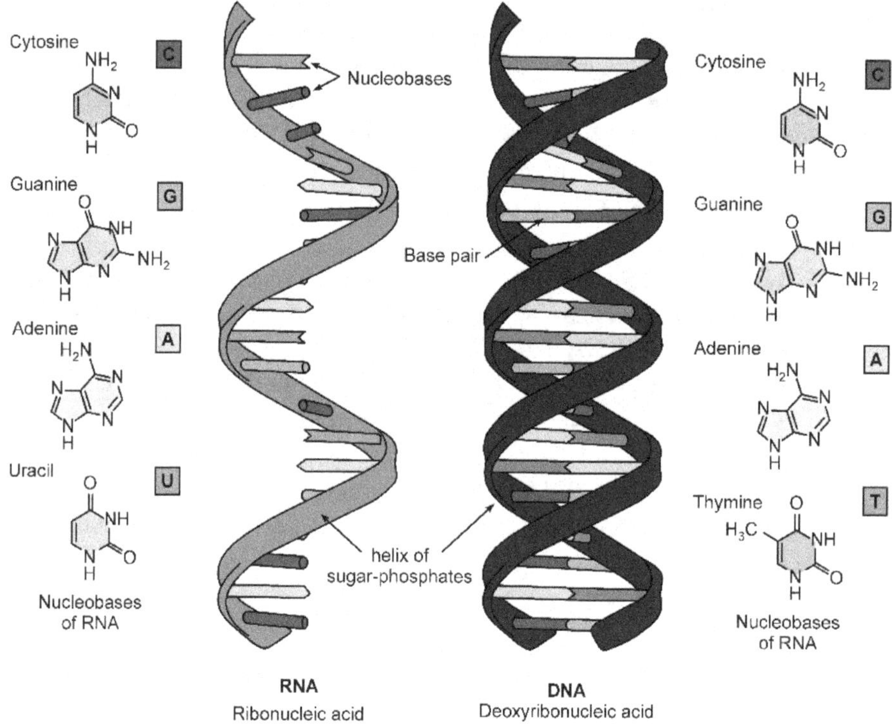

Fig. 5.7 Pictorial representation of difference between RNA and DNA.

Chapter 6

Enzymes

Enzymes are defined as biocatalysts which step up the metabolism and biochemical reactions occurring in our body system. All enzymes are proteins but all proteins are not enzymes in nature.

Properties of Enzymes

1. **Catalytic Property:** - Enzymes increase the metabolic process by acting in small quantities and converting substrate (substance upon which enzyme reacts) into products.

2. **Specificity:** - Enzymes act on specific substrate. An enzymes catalyses one biochemical reaction at a time.

3. **Reversibility:** Enzymes bind reversibly to substrates i.e., a substate bound to enzyme separates after catalysis of biochemical reaction.

4. **Sensitivity to heat, temperature and pH:** - Enzymes are thermolabile in nature and are sensitive to heat, temperature and pH.

IUB and MB Classification of Enzymes

According to **International Union of Biochemistry (IUB)** and **Molecular Biology (MB)** system enzymes are classified into six types:

1. **Oxido-Reductases:** These enzymes are involved in oxidation-reduction reactions between two substrates by involving coenzymes like NAD^+, $NADP^+$ etc. E.g., Alcohol dehydrogenase, cytochrome dehydrogenase, catalase etc.

2. **Transferases:** This class of enzymes helps in transfer of functional groups except hydrogen from one substrate to other substrate. E.g., Phosphorylases, transaminases, acyltransferases etc.

3. **Hydrolases:** These enzymes carry out hydrolysis of various compounds like ester, peptide bonds etc. by the incorporation of water molecules. E.g., Lipase, β-galactosidase, trypsin etc.

4. **Lyases:** These enzymes are involved in removal of functional groups from substrate by process apart from hydrolysis. E.g., Aldolase, different decarboxylase enzymes, fumarase, lyases etc.

5. **Isomerases:** These enzymes carry out isomerization reactions or interconvert isomers (optical, geometric and positional). E.g., Phosphotriose isomerase, epimerases, cis-trans isomerases.

6. **Ligases:** These enzymes help in combining two molecules together and utilises ATP. E.g., Succinate thiokinase, glutamine synthetase, acetyl CoA carboxylase etc.

Factors Affecting Enzyme Activity

1. **Temperature:** Rise in temperature speeds up a biochemical reaction, and decreasing the temperature decelerate a biochemical reaction. Every $10°C$ increase or decrease in temperature directly affects the velocity of an enzyme and it gets double or half respectively. But in case of extreme high temperature enzymes may lose their shape and stop working. This phenomenon is known as denaturing of enzyme.

2. **pH:** Enzymes work at optimum pH range. Alteration of pH out of a range will decrease enzyme activity. However, at extreme pH variation of enzymes may lead to denaturation of enzymes.

3. **Enzyme concentration:** The enzyme velocity is directly proportional to concentration of enzyme. If we increase the concentration of enzyme at constant conditions the velocity also increases to a maximum. But once velocity reaches to maximal value then it is unaffected by further rise in enzyme concentration.

4. **Substrate concentration:** Rise in substrate concentration gradually increases the enzyme velocity but up to a certain point. When velocity is plotted against the substrate concentration, a rectangular hyperbola is attained. The concentration of substrate required to determine half-maximum velocity in enzyme catalysed biochemical reaction can be determined by **Michaelis-Menten Equation**:

$$V = \frac{V_{max}[S]}{Km + [S]}$$

Where, V = Measured velocity

V_{max} = Maximum velocity

$[S]$ = Substrate concentration

K_m = Michaelis-Menten constant (or Brig's and Haldane constant)

K_m implies that 50% of the enzyme is are bound to substrate when $[S]$ or substate concentration is equal to K_m value. It is expressed in moles per litre. The graph plot of substrate-concentration effect on enzyme-velocity is shown in **Fig. 6.1**.

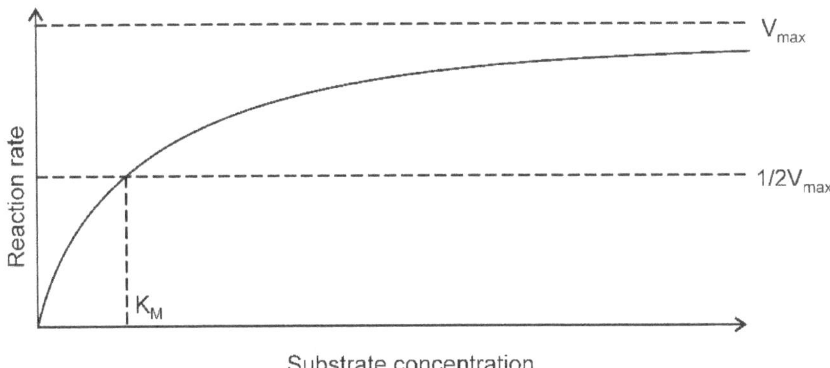

Fig. 6.1 Substrate-concentration effect on enzyme-velocity
(Michaelis-Menten Equation plot).

Mechanism of Action of Enzymes

The enzymes act by attaching the substrates to its active site (main site
present on the enzyme where substrate gets bound and carry out catalysis)
and catalyse the biochemical reaction through which products are formed
and further these products are dissociated from enzyme surface. This leads to
formation of **enzyme-substrate** complex (**Figure 6.2**). Enzymes decrease
the **activation energy** which is required by reactants (substrate and enzyme)
to carry out biochemical or catalysis process.

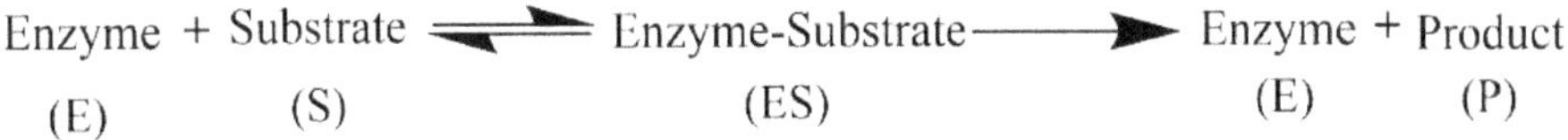

Fig. 6.2 Mechanism of action of enzymes.

The nature of enzymes is remarkably specific. To catalyse a biochemical
reaction, they bind to a specific substrate. Presently two models elaborate the
enzyme specificity: (a) Lock and key model (Fischer's template theory) and
(2) Induced fit model (Koshland's model).

(a) Lock and key model (Fischer's template theory)

This theory was given by the scientist Emil Fischer in 1894 which
highlights the specificity of enzymes. In this model substrate is
considered as key and active site on the enzyme is considered as
lock as shown in figure 6.3. According to this theory a substrate fits
into the specific active site on the enzyme just like a key fit into the
specific lock. This theory also states that a substrate molecule is
complementary in its geometric shape towards the active site of
enzyme.

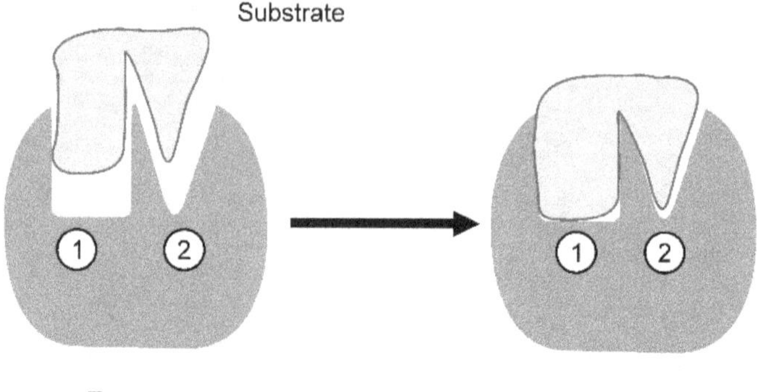

Figure 6.3 Lock and key model

(b) Induced fit model (Koshland's model)

This theory was postulated by the scientist Daniel Koshland in 1958. It states that for best bind fit the active site on the enzyme undergoes a conformational change. In this theory enzymes act as flexible structure as shown in **figure 6.4**. This theory has two main advantages over the lock and key model that this model explains broad specificity and increased reactivity of the substrate towards the active site on the enzyme.

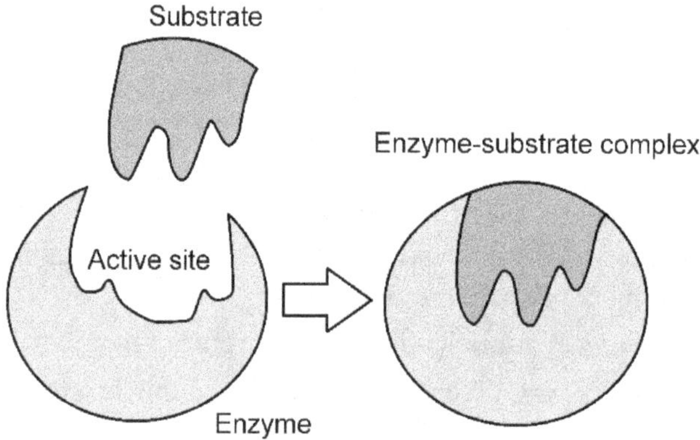

Fig. 6.4 Induced fit model.

Enzyme Inhibitors

Enzyme inhibitors are substances which reduce the enzyme's catalytic activity by binding with the same enzyme. They may be organic or inorganic in nature. The enzyme inhibition is of three main types:

1. Reversible inhibition

2. Irreversible inhibition

3. Allosteric inhibition

   1. Reversible inhibition: In this type of inhibition an enzyme inhibitor binds non-covalently on the enzyme and on the removal of inhibitor, the enzyme inhibition effected can be reversed. It is further subdivided into two main types:

   (a) Competitive inhibition

   (b) Non-competitive inhibition

   (a) **Competitive inhibition:** In this the enzyme inhibitor competes with substrate and binds on the active site of the enzyme but does not bring out any catalysis (**figure 6.5**). In this the value of K_m increases but there is no change in V_{max} value. E.g., Allopurinol competes with hypoxanthine or xanthine substrate for inhibition at the enzyme xanthine oxidase and bring out the decrease in production of uric acid action in gout disease. Another inhibitor dicumarol competes with vitamin K substrate at the vitamin K epoxide reductase enzyme and results in anticoagulant activity.

   (b) **Non-competitive inhibition:** This type of inhibitor binds on the site other than active site in enzymes (**figure 6.5**). This results in impaired enzyme function. In this the K_m value remains unchanged whereas V_{max} is lowered which is the reverse of competitive inhibition. E.g., Heavy metal ions like Ag^+, Pb^{2+}, Hg^{2+} etc. non-competitively inhibit enzymes and bind with cysteinyl sulfhydryl groups.

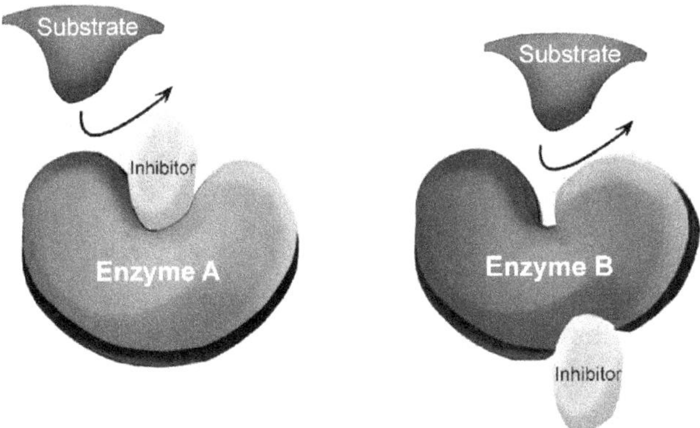

Fig. 6.5 Competitive and non-competitive inhibition.

2. **Irreversible inhibition:** In this type of inhibition the inhibitor irreversibly binds covalently with the enzyme and brings about inactivation of enzyme. E.g., Heavy metals also form covalent bonds with carboxyl groups and brings about irreversible inhibition. Other inhibitors are Iodoacetate (papain and glyceraldehyde 3-phosphate dehydrogenase), Diisopropyl fluorophosphate (DFP) (serine proteases and acetylcholine esterase) and Disulfiram (aldehyde dehydrogenase).

3. **Allosteric inhibition:** It is also known as feedback inhibition. In this inhibition the inhibitor binds to a site other than active site which is known as allosteric site (in Greek: allo-other) on the enzyme and regulates its catalytic activity. Whereas the substrate binds to the active site on the enzyme. The allosteric inhibitors are known as **allosteric modulators** (effector or modifiers). If the positive (+) allosteric inhibitor binds at **allosteric site** then this increases the enzyme activity. Whereas if the negative (-) allosteric effector binds at allosteric site known as **inhibitor site** then this results in enzyme activity inhibition. The allosteric enzymes show sigmoid curve instead of hyperbola curve in contrast to Michaelis-Menten enzymes. E.g., Glucose 6-phosphate is the allosteric inhibitor of the enzyme hexokinase in glycolysis metabolic pathway. Similarly, ATP is the allosteric inhibitor and AMP, ADP are allosteric activator of the enzyme phosphofructokinase in the glycolysis metabolic pathway.

Therapeutic and Pharmaceutical Importance of Enzymes

In pharmaceutical industries enzymes are widely utilised in the number of biochemical transformation reactions like in protection and deprotection of functional groups, acylation, deacylation, hydrolysis, deracemization, esterification, transesterification etc. of various intermediates and compounds in the production of various pharmaceutical products. In pharmaceutical industries enzymes like penicillin acylase and glucose isomerase are utilised in the production of semi synthetic penicillin and fructose syrup.

Enzymes are widely used in the treatment of various diseases. The selective therapeutic applications of enzymes are mentioned here as:

1. The prolactazyme and β-galactosidase enzymes are used to treat lactose intolerance.

2. The collagenase enzyme is prescribed for the treatment of skin ulcer.

3. The streptokinase enzyme is given immediately after a heart attack the patients.

4. The asparaginase enzyme is prescribed for the treatment of leukaemia.

5. The digestive enzymes like papain, lactase, pancrealipase, pepsin etc. are prescribed in digestive disorders.

Chapter 7

Vitamins

The term vitamine (Greek: vita-life) was coined by scientist Funk in 1913. Vitamins may be defined as organic molecules which are essential part of diet and needed in minute quantity for optimum growth of body and maintenance of health. The vitamins are broadly classified into two major classes as fat-soluble vitamins and water-soluble vitamins as shown in **Fig. 7.1**.

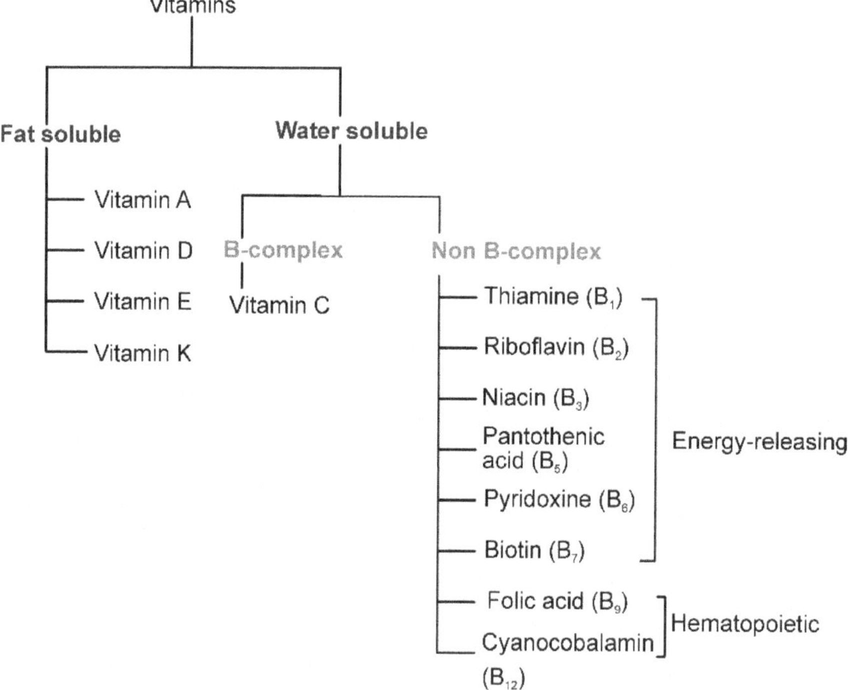

Fig. 7.1 Classification of vitamins.

Fat Soluble Vitamins

Fat soluble vitamins like A, D, E and K gets deposited in adipose tissues. Hence, they are known as fat soluble vitamins.

Vitamin A

Sources: The plant source include yellow vegetables and fruits (carrot, yellow peaches, sweet potato, apricot, and green leafy vegetables). Animal sources include liver, fish liver oil, milk, cheese, and eggs.

Chemical Nature: Vitamin A is also known as retinol **(Fig. 7.2)**. It is a primary alcohol having polyisoprenoid skeleton with β-ionone or cyclohexenyl ring. The precursor of Vitamin A are carotenes (α, β, and γ carotenes). Most effective precursor of Vitamin A is β-carotene.

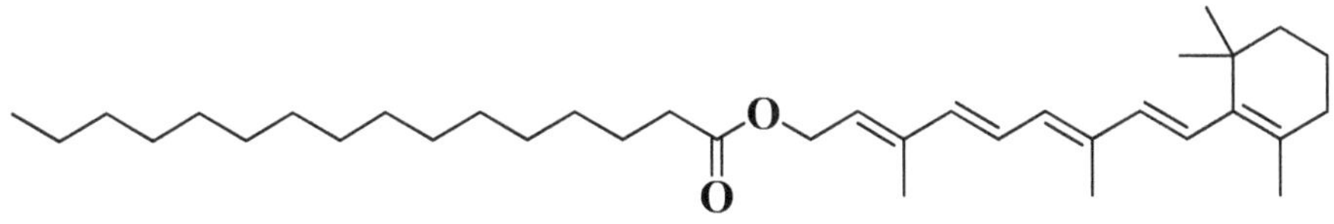

Fig. 7.2 Vitamin A (Retinol).

Coenzyme form: Trans-retinol gets converted to its aldehyde form cis-retinal which is a part of visual pigments known as opsins (rhodopsin and iodopsin).

Recommended dietary requirement:

Infants: 1500 IU

Children: 2000-3000 IU

Adults: 5000 IU

During pregnancy and lactation: 6000-8000 IU

IU = International Unit (1 IU= activity caused by 0.34µg of retinol ester or 0.3µg of retinol or 0.6µg of β-carotene).

Deficiency diseases: Night blindness, xerophthalmia, keratomalacia and hypervitaminosis A.

Functions: Vitamin A performs various functions as:
1. Retinol acts as steroidal hormone and is involved in gene expression.
2. Vitamin A deficiency leads to dry and rough skin (Toad's skin).
3. It helps in reproduction process.
4. Vitamin A prevents from urinary stone formation.
5. The retinal form of vitamin A plays key role in night vision.
6. It helps in development of bones and teeth.

Vitamin D

Sources: Liver, fish, and egg cheese etc. are rich sources of vitamin D.

Chemical Nature: It is also known by the name cholecalciferol **(Fig. 7.3)**. It is steroidal in nature and possess cyclopentanophenanthrene skeleton. It has five forms (D_1, D_2, D_3, D_4, D_5).

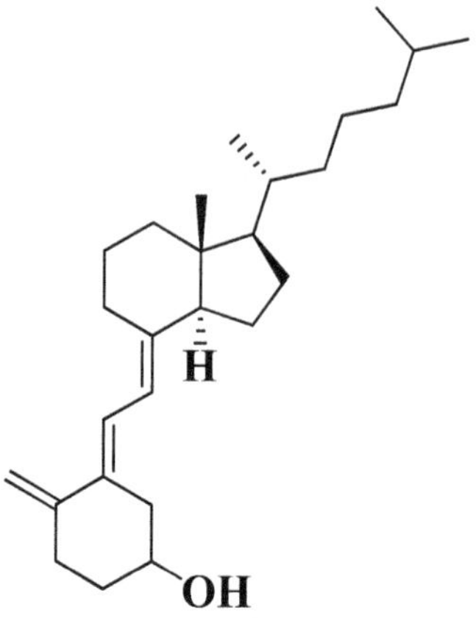

Fig. 7.3 Vitamin D (Cholecalciferol).

Mode of action: The 7-dehydrocholesterol1 gets converted to hormone 25-Dihydroxy cholecalciferol which helps in calcium metabolism regulation through gene expression.

Recommended dietary requirement:

Infants and Children: 400 IU

Adults: Not required in normal condition

During pregnancy and lactation: 500-600 IU

IU = International Unit (1 IU= activity caused by 0.025µg of calciferol)

Deficiency diseases: Vitamin D deficiency causes ricket (in children) and osteomalacia (in adults) characterised by faulty or malformation of bones and deficiency calcium and phosphorous.

Functions:

1. It promotes calcification.
2. It helps in absorption of calcium and phosphorous from intestine.
3. It helps in bone growth and bone healing.

Vitamin E (Antisterility Factor)

Sources: Milk, eggs, meat(muscles), fish and cereals are rich source of vitamin E.

Chemical Nature: It is chemically also known as tocopherol (tokos-child birth and pherein-to bear) **(Fig. 7.4)**. Tocopherol has four forms namely α, β, γ, and δ. Most abundant and biologically active of them is D- α-tocopherol. There chemical structure contains isoprenoid substituted 6-hydroxychromane nucleus.

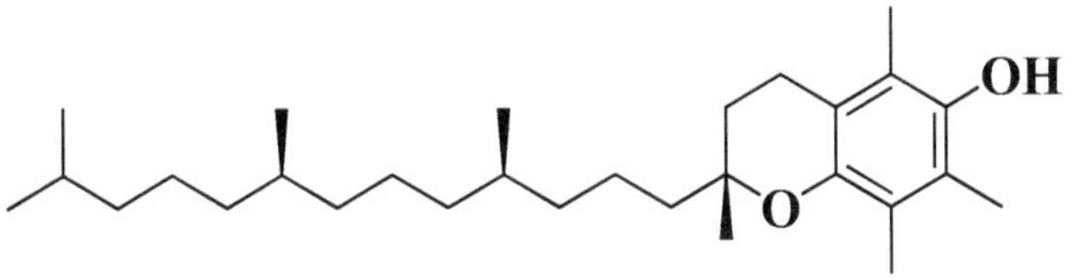

Fig. 7.4 Vitamin E (Tocopherol).

Recommended dietary requirement:

Adults: 30mg

Deficiency diseases: Muscular dystrophy, muscle weakness, mild anaemia with the breakdown of RBC's, sterility in males.

Functions:
1. It acts as natural antioxidant.
2. It synergistically acts with selenium and decreases requirement of each other.
3. It acts as cofactor in electron transport chain (ETC) between 'b' and 'c' cytochromes.

Vitamin K

Sources: Green leafy vegetables, cauliflower, peas, tomato, cereals, egg yolk, liver and cheese are rich source of vitamin K.

Chemical Nature: It is chemically known as phylloquinone **(Fig. 7.5)** in plants and menaquinone **(Fig. 7.6)** in animals and bacteria. It is a naphthoquinone derivative with side chain as polyisoprenoids. It has three forms: vitamin K_1(phylloquinone) and K_2(menaquinone) forms are fat soluble whereas third form K_3(menadione) is water soluble.

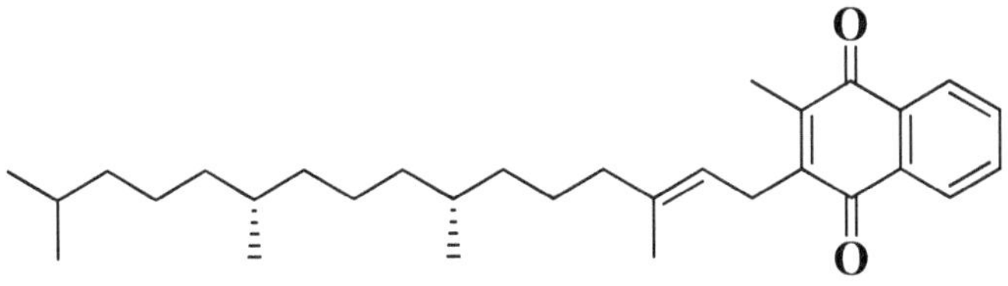

Fig. 7.5 Vitamin K_1 (Phylloquinone or Phytomenadione).

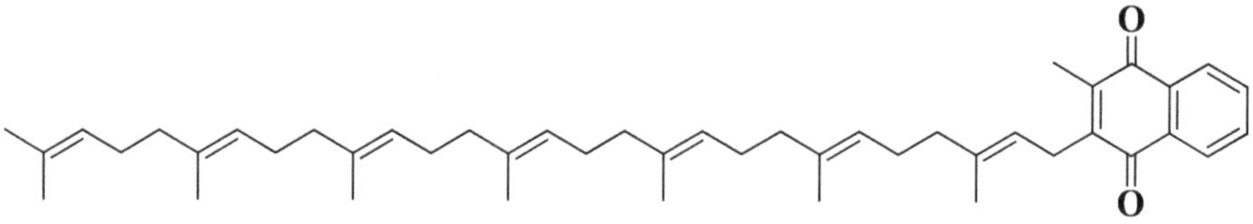

Fig. 7.6 Vitamin K_2 (Menaquinone).

Coenzyme form: Vitamin K serves as coenzyme in the glutamic acid carboxylation.

Recommended dietary requirement:

Adult: 1 mg per day per kg of the body weight.

Deficiency diseases: Vitamin K deficiency causes low prothrombin level and elevation in clotting time which leads to a serious condition known as haemorrhage.

Functions:

1. It helps in biosynthesis of clotting factors II, VII, IX and X.
2. It promotes bone metabolism.
3. It helps in regulation of blood calcium level.

Water Soluble Vitamins

Water soluble vitamins like B-complex and vitamin C does not get deposited in body and they pass through water present in urine. So, they are regularly required by our body in diet.

Vitamin B₁ (Antiberiberi factor, Aneurine)

Sources: Cereals and grains(unrefined), liver, heart and kidney.

Chemical Nature: It is chemically known as thiamine **(Fig. 7.7)** and is a substituted pyrimidine i.e., 2,5-dimethyl-6-aminopyrimidine joined with substituted thiazole ring and methylene bridge.

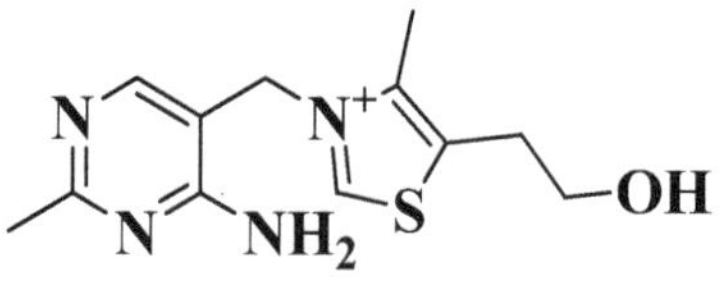

Fig. 7.7 Vitamin B_1 (Thiamine).

Coenzyme form: It is precursor of coenzyme of central metabolic pathways thiamine diphosphate (ThDP) which helps in glucose oxidation.

Recommended dietary requirement

Infants: 0.3-0.5mg

Children: 0.7-1.2 mg

Adults:

Male:1.5 mg

Female: 1.2 mg

Deficiency diseases: Beriberi (It is of three types: dry, wet and infantile beriberi)

Functions:

1. It helps the body's cells to convert carbohydrates into energy.
2. It plays a significant role in muscle contraction and conduction of nerve signals.

Vitamin B$_2$

Sources: Milk, liver, kidney, heart, green vegetables and germinating seeds.

Chemical Nature: It chemically also known as riboflavin **(Fig. 7.8)** and comprises of isoalloxazine ring joined to sugar alcohol-ribitol.

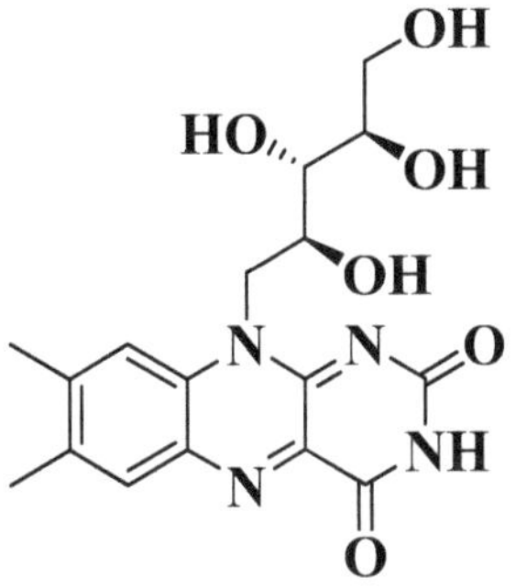

Fig. 7.8 Vitamin B$_2$ (Riboflavin).

Coenzyme form: Flavin mononucleotide (FMN) and adenine dinucleotide (FAD)

Recommended dietary requirement:

Infants: 0.4-0.6mg

Children: 0.8-1.2 mg

Adults: 1.2-1.7mg

During pregnancy and lactation: 0.3-0.6mg is additionally required

Deficiency diseases: Angular stomatitis (fissures formed at the angle of mouth), Cheilosis (red epithelium zone formation at the closure line of lips), Glossitis (inflammation of tongue)

Functions:

1. It works with the other B-complex vitamins and is important for body growth.

2. It promotes red blood cell production.

3. It helps in the release of energy from proteins.

Vitamin B₃ (Pellagra Preventive Factor)

Sources: Unrefined cereals and grains(rice), yeast, milk, egg, tomato, fruits, and green vegetables etc.

Chemical Nature: Chemically it is known as niacin or nicotinic acid **(Fig. 7.9)** and is a pyridine derivative in nature.

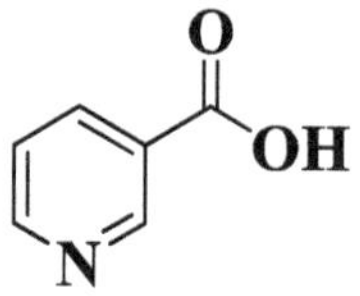

Fig. 7.9 Vitamin B₃ (Niacin or Nicotinic Acid).

Coenzyme form: Nicotinamide adenine dinucleotide (NAD) and nicotinamide adenine dinucleotide phosphate (NADP)

Recommended dietary requirement:

Infants: 5-8 mg

Children: 9-16 mg

Adults:

Male: 16-20mg

Female: 12-16mg

During pregnancy 3mg and during lactation: 7mg is additionally required

Deficiency disease: Pellagra (Symptoms are dermatitis, dementia and diarrhoea).

Functions:

1. NAD and NADP acts as coenzymes for most of the oxidoreductase enzymes.
2. NAD is a part of ETC or respiratory chain.
3. Niacin decreases plasma cholesterol.

Vitamin B_{12}

Sources: Liver, kidney. Meat, fish and eggs.

Chemical Nature: It is also known as cyanocobalamin **(Fig. 7.10)**. Its structure is comprised of four substituted pyrrole rings surrounded by central cobalt atom known as corrin ring system. Below the corrin ring a compound 5,6-dimethyl benzimidazole riboside is attached to one end of cobalt atom and another end to ribose with the help of phosphate and aminopropanol.

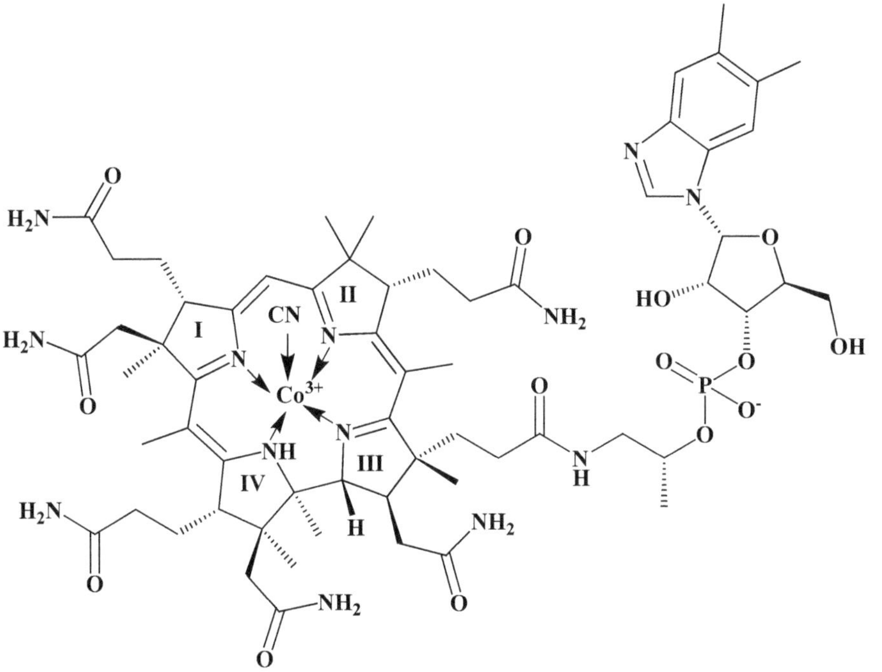

Fig. 7.10 Vitamin B_{12} (Cyanocobalamin).

Coenzyme form: Methyl cobalamin and 5-deoxyadenosylcobalamin

Recommended dietary requirement:

Infants: $0.3\mu g$

Children: $1\text{-}2\mu g$

Adults: $3\mu g$

During pregnancy and lactation $4\mu g$ is required.

Deficiency diseases: Pernicious anaemia (caused due to decreased absorption and lack of intrinsic factor).

Functions

1. Vitamin B_{12} is required in the formation of red blood cells and DNA.

2. It helps in proper functioning and growth of brain and nerve cells.

3. It gets bound to the protein in the foods we eat.

Biotin or Vitamin B₇ or Vitamin H (Anti-egg White Injury Factor)

Sources: Liver, kidney, yeast, milk, fruits, egg yolk, vegetables, and yeast.

Chemical Nature: Biotin **(Fig. 7.11)** is a imidazole derivative having sulphur atom.

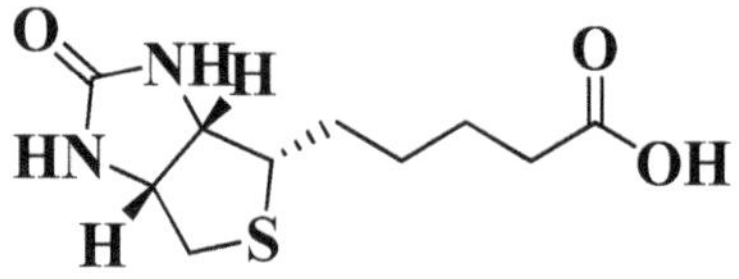

Fig. 7.11 Biotin.

Coenzyme form: Coenzyme R and biotin itself acts as coenzyme for five carboxylase enzymes.

Recommended dietary requirement: 50-60µg

Deficiency diseases: The raw egg white contains avidin. When we consume raw egg white the avidin gets fused with biotin and blocks its absorption in the body leading to biotin deficiency with symptoms as loss of hair, depression, muscle pain, retarded growth etc.

Functions

1. Biotin is needed to metabolize carbohydrates, fats, and amino acids.

2. It strengthens hair and nails, and is ingredient of many cosmetic products for hair and skin.

Folic Acid

Sources: Green leafy vegetables, yeast, and liver.

Chemical Nature: Folic acid structure **(Fig. 7.12)** consists of pteridine base joined with p-aminobenzoic acid and glutamic acid. It is present in liver as Penta glutamate.

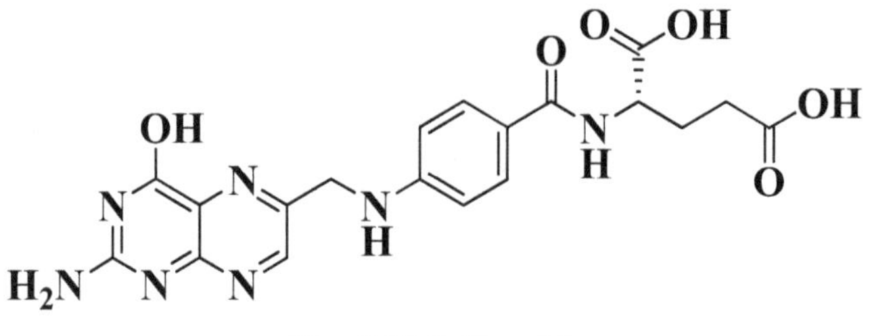

Fig. 7.12 Folic acid.

Coenzyme form: Tetrahydro folic acid

Recommended dietary requirement:

Infants: 50µg

Children: 100-300µg

Adults: 400µg

During pregnancy and lactation 600-800µg is required.

Deficiency diseases: Megaloblastic anaemia

Functions:

1. It is involved metabolism of one carbon moieties.
2. It plays key role in mental and emotional health.
3. It helps in the formation of genetic material i.e., DNA and RNA.

Vitamin C

Sources: Citrus fruits (amla, tomato, lemon, berries, and grapes etc.)

Chemical Nature: It is chemically known as ascorbic acid **(Figure 7.13)** which is an enediol lactone. It resembles to L-glucose and is oxidised readily to dehydroascorbic acid.

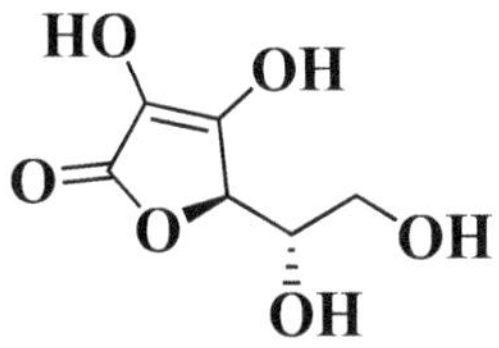

Fig. 7.13 Vitamin C (Ascorbic acid).

Coenzyme form: It is used as coenzyme in hydroxylation of proline in collagen which promotes wound healing.

Recommended dietary requirement:

Infants: 30mg

Children: 40mg

Adults: 50-70mg

During pregnancy and lactation: 60-80mg

Deficiency diseases: Scurvy

Functions:

1. It is strong reducing agent.
2. It helps in wound healing by promoting the hydroxylation of proline in collagen.

3. It required in biosynthesis of bile acids.

4. It is required in absorption and metabolism of iron.

The brief summary of vitamin sources and deficiency diseases are given in **Table 7.1**.

Table 7.1 Table containing summary of vitamin sources and deficiency diseases.

Sr. No.	Vitamin	Solubility	Source	Deficiency Diseases
1.	Vitamin A	Fat	Carrot, yellow peaches, sweet potato, apricot, and green leafy vegetables, liver, fish liver oil, milk, cheese, and egg	Liver, fish liver oil, milk, cheese, and eggs
2.	Vitamin D	Fat	Liver, fish, egg, and cheese	Ricket (in children) and osteomalacia (in adults)
3.	Vitamin E (Antisterility factor)	Fat	Milk, eggs, meat(muscles), fish and cereals	Muscular dystrophy, muscle weakness, and mild anaemia
4.	Vitamin K	Fat	Green leafy vegetables, cauliflower, peas, tomato, cereals, egg yolk, liver and cheese	Haemorrhage
5.	Vitamin B_1 (Antiberiberi factor, Aneurine)	Water	Cereals and grains(unrefined), liver, heart and kidney	Beriberi
6.	Vitamin B_2	Water	Milk, liver, kidney, heart, green vegetables and germinating seeds.	Angular stomatitis, Cheilosis, Glossitis
7.	Vitamin B_3 (Pellagra Preventive Factor)	Water	Unrefined cereals and grains(rice), yeast, milk, egg, tomato, fruits, and green vegetables	Pellagra
8.	Vitamin B_{12}	Water	Liver, kidney. Meat, fish and eggs.	Pernicious anaemia
9.	Biotin or Vitamin B_7 or Vitamin H (Anti-egg White Injury Factor)	Water	Liver, kidney, yeast, milk, fruits, egg yolk, vegetables, yeast	Biotin deficiency with symptoms as loss of hair, depression, muscle pain, retarded growth etc.
10.	Folic Acid	Water	Green leafy vegetables, yeast, liver	Megaloblastic anaemia
11.	Vitamin C	Water	Citrus fruits (amla, tomato, lemon, berries, grapes etc.)	Scurvy

Chapter 8

Metabolism

Metabolism is defined as the involvement of biochemical reactions assuring the living state of organism through the proper functioning of cells. It is of two types:

1. Catabolism – splitting of larger molecules to smaller one to gain energy
2. Anabolism – the fusion of all molecules required by the body cells

Metabolism is associated with the nutrition and the accessibility of nutrients. Bioenergetics is defined as the series of biochemical or metabolic pathways through which the body cells gain energy. Energy generation is the essential part of metabolism process.

Metabolism of Carbohydrates

Carbohydrate metabolism is an essential biochemical step that assures a constant energy supply to the living body cells. Glucose is considered as the important carbohydrate which can be splitted through glycolysis pathway and then introduced to the Kreb's cycle and oxidative phosphorylation to produce ATP.

Glycolysis

Glycolysis (glycol-sugar, lysis-breakdown) is defined as splitting of sugars with the release of energy. This pathway was elucidated by two biochemists Embden and Meyerhof in 1940 therefore it is also known as Embden-Meyerhof pathway (E.M. pathway). In this process a six-carbon containing carbohydrate i.e., glucose or glycogen splits into three carbon atoms containing molecule pyruvate or lactate with the generation of ATP.

Salient features of glycolysis:

Glycolysis is a universal pathway as it takes place in all the cells of living body.

The enzymes responsible for the function of this pathway are present in cytostome part of body cells.

It occurs in both aerobic and anaerobic conditions and the end products of this pathway are different in both the conditions i.e., pyruvate and lactate respectively.

Tissues like cornea, lens and erythrocytes lack mitochondria. So, glycolysis is the main energy supply pathways in these tissues.

It is an important pathway in brain which requires energy in uninterruptable manner through glucose. The glucose further gets oxidized to CO_2 and H_2O with the help of glycolysis.

Reactions of Glycolysis

Glycolysis reactions are split into three stages:

(a) Energy investment or priming phase

(b) Splitting phase

(c) Energy generation phase

(a) Energy investment or priming phase:

1. In the first step enzyme hexokinase or glucokinase (both of them are isoenzymes) phosphorylates glucose molecule present in cytoplasm of cell. This biochemical reaction takes place in presence of Mg^{2+} ions with conversion of ATP to ADP. The resultant product is called as glucose 6-phosphate(G6P).

2. In the next step phosphohexose isomerase enzyme and Mg^{2+} ions isomerize G6P into its isomer form fructose 6-phosphate (F6P).

3. Further, phosphofructokinase (PFK) enzymes phosphorylate F6P to fructose 1,6-bisphosphate in an irreversible manner.

Splitting phase

4. Fructose 1,6-bisphosphate breaks down two three-carbon containing compounds i.e., glyceraldehyde 3-phosphate and dihydroxyacetone phosphate in presence of enzyme aldolase or fructose 1,6-bisphosphate aldolase. That why this pathway is termed as "glycolysis".

5. The phosphotriose isomerase enzyme helps in catalysis of inter-conversion of glyceraldehyde 3-phosphate and dihydroxyacetone phosphate in an irreversible manner. Both these two compounds (glyceraldehyde 3-phosphate and dihydroxyacetone phosphate) are produced through a single glucose molecule.

Energy generation phase

6. In this phase glyceraldehyde-3-phosphate gets converted to energy rich molecule 1,3-Bisphosphoglycerate due to the existence of enzyme glyceraldehyde-3-phosphate dehydrogenase. In this step

there is generation of NADH. The glyceraldehyde-3-phosphate enzyme is inhibited by compounds arsenate and iodoacetate.

7. Further the compound 1,3-phosphoglycerate gets converted to 3-phosphoglycerate with the generation of ATP molecule in presence of enzyme phosphoglycerate. This reaction is also irreversible in nature. This step involves synthesis of ATP from the substrate without including the electron transport chain process. So, this is a best example of substrate level phosphorylation.

8. In the next step the compound 3-phosphoglycerate gets converted to 2-phosphoglycerate by the enzyme phosphoglycerate mutase. This step is an excellent illustration of isomerization reaction.

9. Further the compound phosphoenol pyruvate (energy rich compound) is produced from 2-phosphoglycerate in presence of enolase enzyme and Mg^{2+}/Mn^{2+} ions. The enolase enzyme is inhibited by the fluoride.

10. Finally, the energy rich phosphoenol pyruvate compound gets converted to pyruvate compound in presence of enzyme pyruvate kinase and further pyruvate gets changed to lactate in presence of lactate dehydrogenase enzyme respectively with the formation of ATP from ADP. This reaction step is irreversible in nature and also example of substrate level phosphorylation. The steps involved in glycolysis pathway are shown in **Fig. 8.1** and total number of ATP generated or utilized during the pathway are summarized in **Table 8.1**.

Significance of Conversion of Pyruvate to Lactate

The erythrocytes lack mitochondria which is the main site for aerobic respiration. The glycolysis pathway produces lactate in erythrocytes. During vigorous exercise skeletal muscles having limited oxygen supply also undergo glycolysis to meet energy demand. Even other parts of body like retina, brain, skin, gastrointestinal tract and renal medulla are dependent on glycolysis to gain energy.

Table 8.1 ATP synthesis in Glycolysis pathway

Enzyme/method involved	No. of ATP
Glyceraldehyde 3-phosphate dehydrogenase (2 NADH, ETC, Oxidative phosphorylation)	6
Phosphoglycerate kinase (Substrate level phosphorylation)	2
Pyruvate kinase (Substrate level phosphorylation)	2
Two ATP are utilized in the reactions catalyzed by hexokinase and phosphofructokinase enzymes	−2
Net ATP generated in glycolysis pathway (Aerobic conditions)	**8**

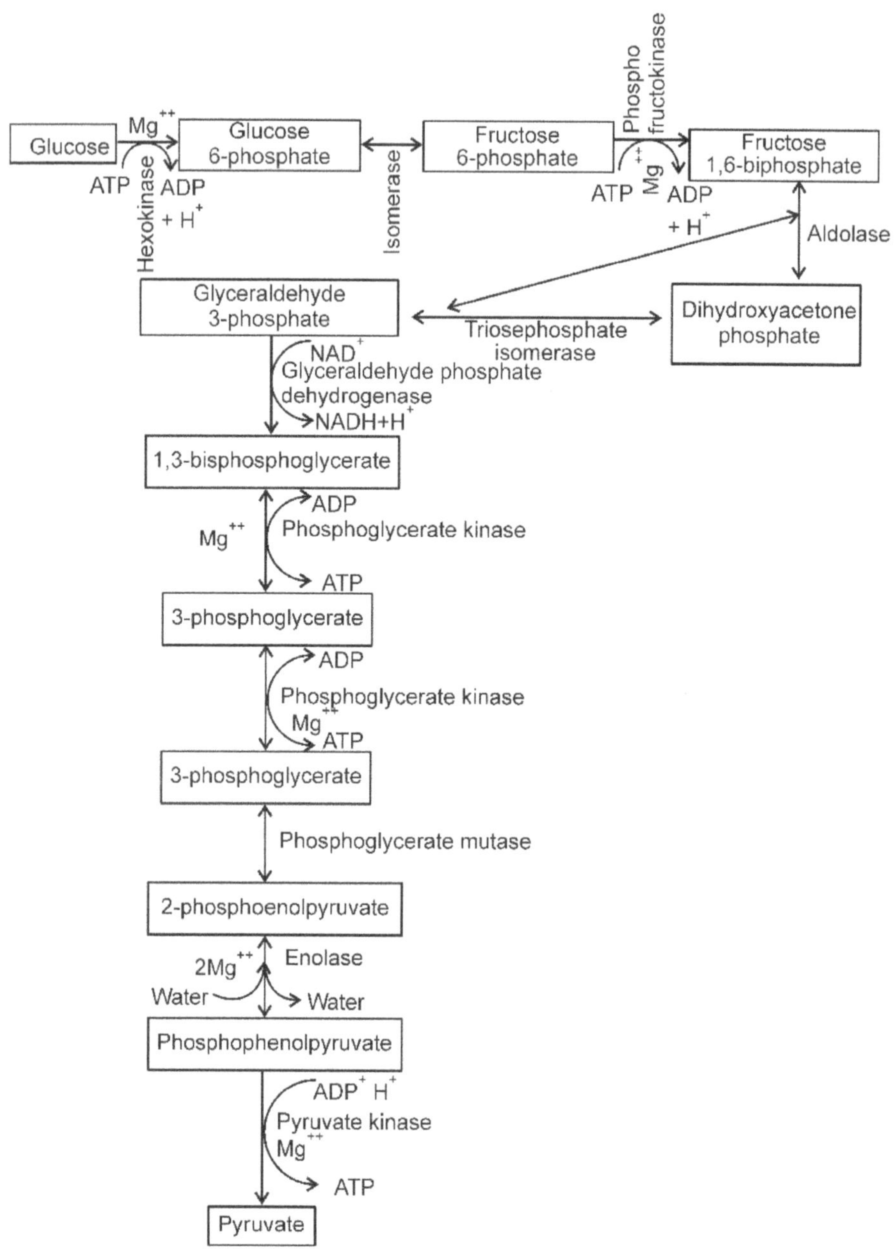

Fig. 8.1 Steps involved in glycolysis pathway.

TCA Cycle and Glycogen Metabolism

The TCA cycle (tricarboxylic acid cycle) is also known by the names, citric acid and Kreb's Cycle (name in the honour of its discoverer Hans Adolf Krebs in 1937). It is a major metabolic pathway which synthesizes 65-70% of the ATP in body. Kreb's cycle oxidises acetyl CoA to CO_2 and H_2O. This cycle is named TCA because it involves three carboxylic acid derivatives namely citrate, cis-aconitate and isocitrate.

The TCA cycle is a central metabolic pathway which combines almost all the other metabolic pathways either directly or indirectly. Because this pathway yields intermediates for generation of molecules like glucose, heme, and amino acids etc. So, finally we can say that TCA cycle is the oxidative pathway for complete metabolism of carbohydrates, amino acids and lipids.

The enzymes involved in TCA cycle are present in mitochondrial matrix of the cell. The ETC (electron transport chain) assembly is also present in the mitochondria which connects both the pathways closely leading to the production of ATP by oxidative phosphorylation process. The TCA cycle is an open cycle and should not be considered as closed cycle because many intermediates formed in this cycle also participated in other metabolic pathways. The overview of TCA cycle is given in **Fig. 8.2**.

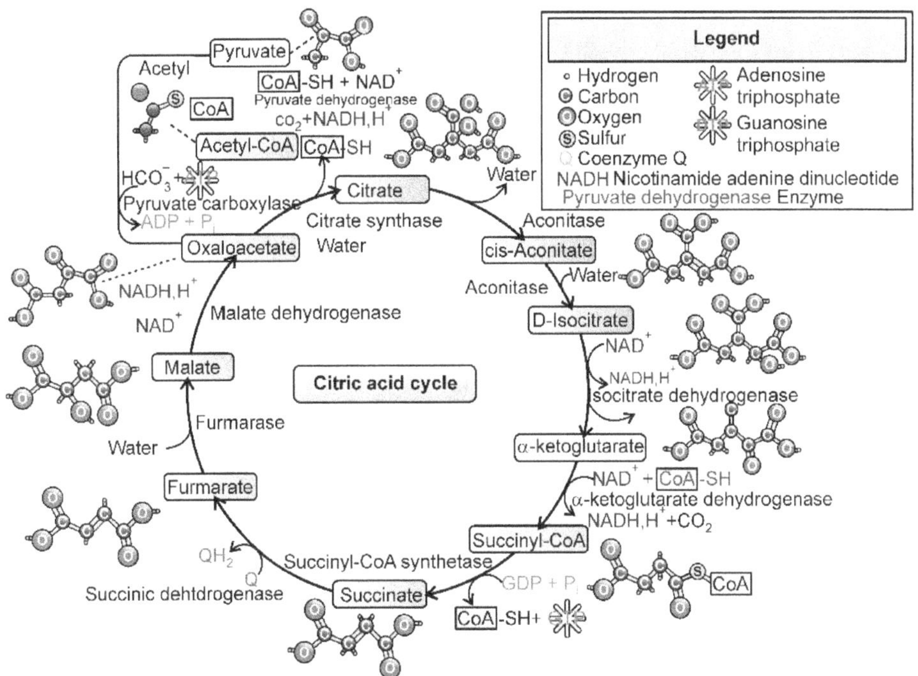

Fig. 8.2 TCA cycle or Citric acid cycle or Kreb's cycle.

Reactions of TCA Cycle

1. In the first step pyruvate gets converted to acetyl CoA in presence of enzyme pyruvate dehydrogenase. The acetyl CoA further combines with oxaloacetate to form citrate in presence of enzyme citrate synthase.

2. In the next step aconitase enzyme isomerises the citrate to isocitrate. The reaction follows two steps i.e., dehydration and hydration with the formation of cis-aconitate as intermediate.

3. Further the isocitrate compound gets converted to oxalosuccinate and then to α-ketoglutarate in presence of enzyme isocitrate dehydrogenase (ICD). This step follows oxidative decarboxylation process. There is generation of NADPH and release of carbon dioxide in this step.

4. In this step α-ketoglutarate gets converted to succinyl CoA with the help of oxidative decarboxylation process. This conversion reaction is catalysed by α-ketoglutarate dehydrogenase enzyme complex. The cofactors upon which enzyme complex is dependent include TPP, lipoamide, NAD+, FAD and CoA.

5. In the next step enzyme succinate thiokinase converts succinyl CoA to succinate with the phosphorylation of GDP to GTP followed by conversion to ATP. The reaction follows substrate level phosphorylation process. The enzyme responsible for conversion of GTP to ATP is nucleoside diphosphate kinase.

6. Further enzyme succinate dehydrogenase oxidises succinate to fumarate with the generation of $FADH_2$.

7. In this second last step fumarate gets converted to malate in presence of enzyme fumarase with the inclusion of H_2O molecule.

8. In the final step, oxidation of malate to oxaloacetate takes place with the generation of NADH. This final generated compound oxaloacetate further couples with acetyl CoA to carry on this TCA cycle.

Energetics of TCA Cycle (Table 8.2)

- The oxidation of three NADH with oxidative phosphorylation (coupled with ETC) results in the generation of **nine ATP**.
- The $FADH_2$ results in generation of **two ATP**.
- There is formation of **an ATP** from one substrate level phosphorylation.
- Therefore, a total of **twelve ATP** is generated from one acetyl CoA.

Table 8.2 Energetics of TCA cycle

Enzyme/method involved	No. of ATP
Oxidation of three NADH with oxidative phosphorylation	9
FADH₂	2
Substrate level phosphorylation	1
Total	**12**

Regulation of Blood Glucose

The blood glucose level of a normal person is 80 to 120 mg/dL but due to excessive diet intake or vigorous exercise there is fluctuation in blood glucose level. This fluctuation in blood glucose level occurs due to variety of hormonally triggered changes in the metabolism of several organs.

Carbohydrate metabolism is regulated by the hormones like insulin, glucagon, epinephrine or adrenaline, glucocorticoids, thyroxine, ACTH and growth hormone etc. Each one of these hormones are discussed here and outline is shown in **Fig. 8.3**.

Insulin: Insulin is a peptide hormone secreted by β-cells of islets of Langerhans of pancreas. It regulates the metabolism of carbohydrates and fats. After a carbohydrate rich meal, the glucose enters the blood stream from the intestine resulting in increased blood flow. The elevated concentration of blood glucose stimulates the release of insulin which lowers the increased blood glucose level. Insulin lowers the increased blood glucose i.e., hyperglycemia by promoting glycolysis and spread the uptake of glucose by tissues via glycogenesis favoring the storage of fuels as glycogen and triacyl glycerides while it suppresses glycogenolysis and gluconeo-genesis.

Glucagon: It is secreted by α-cells of islets of Langerhans of pancreas. It shows activity opposite to that of insulin. When the concentration of insulin and indirectly glucose in the blood stream falls to low then glucagon is released from pancreas and it causes the conversion of glycogen to glucose by promoting glycogenolysis and gluconeogenesis. When glucagon binds to the glucagon receptors, the liver cells convert glycogen into individual glucose molecules and release them into the blood stream. Glucagon also regulates the rate of glucose production through lipolysis.

Epinephrine/adrenaline: This hormone is secreted by adrenal medulla. Its effect is mediated through the hypothalamus in response to low blood glucose. It acts both on muscle and liver to bring about glycogenolysis by increasing phosphorylase activity. The end product is glucose in liver and lactate in muscle. The net outcome is that epinephrine increases blood glucose level.

Glucocorticoids: These hormones are produced by adrenal cortex. Gluco-corticoids stimulate protein metabolism and gluconeogenesis by increasing the activity of glucose-6-phosphatase and fructose-1,6-bisphosphatase. The glucose used by extrahepatic tissues is inhibited by glucocorticoids. The overall effect is to increase the blood glucose concentration.

Thyroxine: This hormone is secreted by of thyroid gland. It increases blood glucose level with stimulation of hepatic glycogenolysis and gluconeogenesis metabolic processes.

ACTH and GH: ACTH and GH stands for adrenocorticotropic hormone and growth hormone respectively. Both these hormones are secreted by anterior pituitary gland. The glucose uptake by specific tissues i.e., muscle, adipose tissue etc. is reduced by growth hormone. The ACTH also reduces utilization of glucose. So, the net result of both these hormones is hyperglycemia.

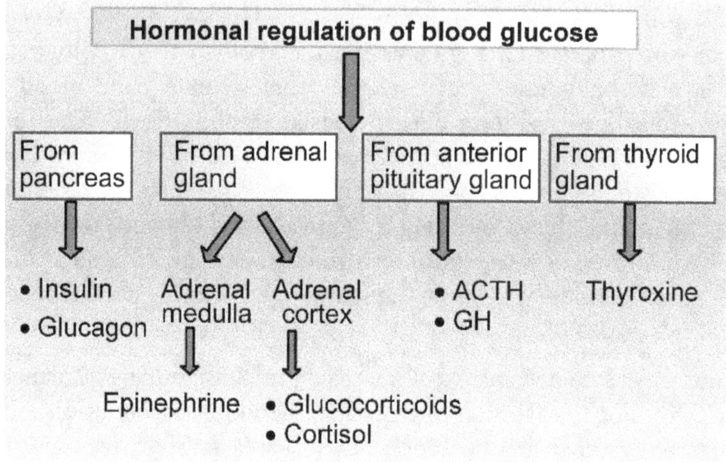

Fig. 8.3 Hormonal regulation of blood glucose.

Diseases Related to Abnormal Metabolism of Carbohydrates

Diabetes Mellitus (DM):

As per WHO, diabetes mellitus (DM) is defined as a chronic metabolic disorder identified by chronic hyperglycemia/ glycosuria with disturbance of carbohydrates, fat and protein metabolism. The classification of blood sugar level is shown in the **table 8.3.**

Table 8.3 Classification of blood sugar level

Blood sugar level classification	Fasting blood sugar level	After meals blood sugar level
Normal Person	70-100 mg/dL	70-140 mg/dL
Prediabetic Person	101-125 mg/dL	141-200 mg/dL
Diabetic Person	125mg/dL and above	200 mg/dL and above

This is due to deficiency or absence of insulin or rarely the impairment of insulin activity i.e., insulin resistance causing varying degrees of disruption of carbohydrates and fat metabolism. Diabetes is the major cause of adult blindness, renal failure and cardiac diseases.

Types

DM is divided into two main types:

1. Type-I (IDDM)
2. Type-II (NIDDM)
3. Type-III (Gestational DM)

Type-I(IDDM): It is also known as insulin dependent diabetes mellitus. It is characterized by auto-immune destruction or deficiency of β-cells of islets of Langerhans of pancreas. It occurs in children and young adults and the onset is usually sudden. It is traditionally termed as juvenile diabetes. This type comprises up to 10% cases of DM. The most common cause of type-I is an autoimmune reaction has occurred in which autoantibodies destroy β-cells. Type-I diabetics cannot produce insulin; hence they should get insulin through insulin injections.

Type-II (NIDDM): It is also known as non-insulin dependent diabetes mellitus (NIDDM). This is the most common form of DM accounting about 90% cases of DM. There is enough insulin but cells become resistant to insulin over a long period of time. Liver, adipose tissue and muscle do not respond properly to it and this leads to uncontrolled production of glucose by liver and decreased uptake of glucose by muscle and adipose tissue. It is usually diagnosed after 30-40 yrs of age. It is called late onset because it appears late in life.

Type-III (Gestational DM): It is often known as gestational diabetes mellitus. It is defined as glucose intolerance which is first recognized during pregnancy, gestational diabetes complicates about 7% of all pregnancies and it may disappear after delivery. GDM may damage the health of fetus or mother and 40% of women with GD develop type-II diabetes later in life.

Other Disorders

Galactosemia: It is an inherited disorder of galactose metabolism. Mainly three enzymes involved in galactose metabolism are: galactose 1-phosphate uridyl transferase, galactokinase and UDP galactose 4-epimerase. Galactosemia is caused due to the deficiency of any one of the above three enzymes. The symptoms include cataract (due to accumulation of polyol or galactitol which is reduced form of galactose), liver failure and degradation of mental health.

Renal glycosuria: This is characterised by excretion of glucose in urine due to defective renal tubular absorption of glucose. The blood glucose level in this disease is normal.

Essential Fructosuria: In this disorder, fructose is found in urine due to the deficiency of fructokinase enzyme.

Essential Pentosuria: A inherited disease usually identified by L-xylulose excretion in urine due to the deficiency of L-xylulose reductase enzyme.

Glycogen Storage Diseases (GSD): The glycogen storage diseases are metabolic defects which deal with the generation and deterioration of glycogen. These diseases are identified by accumulation of normal or abnormal type of glycogen in one or more tissues. These include Von Gierke's disease (type I glycogenosis, Pomp's disease, Cori's disease (limit dextrinosis or Forbe's disease) etc.

Metabolism of Lipids

The generation and degradation of lipids inside the cells is known as lipid metabolism. It includes either lysis or deposition of lipids for energy. The lipids are retrieved through food consumption and then absorbed. However, liver also synthesise fats. Very small amount of fat is required by our body for the synthesis of essential fatty acids, for the absorption of fat-soluble vitamins, source of energy (1gm fat gives 9.1 calories). The end products of fatty acid metabolism include CO_2, H_2O and ATP.

Lipolysis

Lipolysis is defined as breakdown of fats inside the body in presence of enzymes and water or through hydrolysis. It mainly takes place in adipose tissues or fatty tissues.

Salient features of lipolysis:

- It involves triglyceride hydrolysis into glycerol and three molecules of fatty acid.

- Three lipase enzymes are used in this process i.e., hormone sensitive lipase, diacyl glycerol lipase and monoacyl glycerol lipase.

- The diacyl glycerol lipase and monoacyl glycerol lipase are responsible for hydrolysis of diacyl and monoacylglycerols to fatty acids and glycerols in a rapid and exhaustive manner.

- The action of hormone sensitive lipase on adipose tissue is controlled by hormones like glucagon, epinephrine, norepinephrine and adrenocorticotrophic.

- These hormones stimulate lipolysis and activate adenylate cyclase which further boosts up the generation of cAMP (cyclic adenosine monophosphate)

- This leads to activation of protein kinase A which further activates other lipases present inside the adipose tissue.

- The fate of glycerol and fatty acids after lipolysis is diffusion through plasma membrane into the blood stream.

β-oxidation of Fatty Acid (Palmitic Acid)

β-oxidation is a metabolic process through fatty acids get oxidized in our body. The oxidation generally takes place on the β-carbon atom in a fatty acid hence the pathway is known as β-oxidation of fatty acids. The final outcome of this pathway is sequential cleavage of a two-carbon fragment and acetyl CoA.

The β-oxidation of fatty acids is divided into three phases:

I. Fatty acid activation (occurs in the cytosol)

II. Fatty acids transportation into mitochondria

III. β-Oxidation proper in the mitochondrial matrix

I. Fatty acid activation

In the first stage activation of fatty acids to acyl CoA occurs through thiokinases or acyl CoA synthetases enzymes. This is a two-step reaction and involves ATP, coenzyme A and Mg^{2+} ions. In this step two high energy phosphate compounds are used as involving ATP to get converted to pyrophosphate (PPi).

II. Fatty acids transportation into mitochondria

The fatty acids cannot cross through inner mitochondrial membrane. Therefore, a special transport system known as carnitine carrier system or carnitine shuttle helps fatty acids to travel from cytosol to mitochondria. This process generally involves four stages:

1. The acyl group present in acyl CoA gets shifted to carnitine (β-hydroxy γ-trimethyl aminobutyrate) with the help of enzyme carnitine acyltransferase I. This enzyme is found on the outer part of the inner mitochondrial membrane.

2. In the next step, transportation of acyl-carnitine through membrane to mitochondrial matrix takes place with the help of a specific carrier protein.

3. Further the Carnitine acyl transferase II (an enzyme present in the inner facial of the inner mitochondrial membrane) changes acyl-carnitine to acyl CoA.

4. In the last stage the carnitine liberated restores to cytosol for recycle.

III. β-Oxidation proper

The β-oxidation cycle follows a sequence of four step reactions resulting in release of a two carbon unit-acetyl CoA.

1. Oxidation: With the help of enzyme acyl CoA dehydrogenase (an FAD-dependent flavoenzyme) the compound acyl CoA follows dehydrogenation reaction. This results in formation of a double bond among αand β carbons or between 2 and 3 carbons.

2. Hydration: In this step there is formation of β-hydroxyacyl CoA compound due to the hydration of double bond caused by the enzyme enoyl CoA hydratase.

3. Oxidation: Due to catalysis of enzyme β-hydroxyacyl CoA dehydrogenase there is formation of compound β-ketoacyl CoA through oxidation process. The NADH gets formed during this reaction.

4. Cleavage: In this final step, the enzyme β-ketoacyl CoA thiolase or thiolase carry out a thiolytic cleavage resulting in release of two carbon containing compounds namely acetyl CoA and acyl CoA. The acyl CoA formed reenters and undergo β-oxidation cycle. This cycle keeps on repeating till complete oxidation of fatty acid occurs. The general β-oxidation pathway and β-oxidation of palmitic acid pathway are shown in figures 8.4 and 8.5 respectively. The energetics of β-oxidation of palmitic acid is shown in Fig. 8.4.

Table 8.4 Energetics of β-oxidation of palmitic acid

Mechanism	ATP Yield
I. β-Oxidation (Seven Cycles)	
7 FADH₂ (Each FADH₂ oxidized by ETC (Electron transport chain) yields two ATP)	14
7 NADH (Each NADH oxidized by ETC (Electron transport chain) yields three ATP)	21
II. From acetyl CoA (eight)	
Each acetyl CoA oxidized by Kreb's cycle or TCA cycle gives 12 ATP	96
Total energy (from 1 mole of palmitoyl CoA)	**131**
Energy used during activation step in the generation of palmitoyl CoA	-2
Net yield (for 1molecule of palmitic acid)	**129**

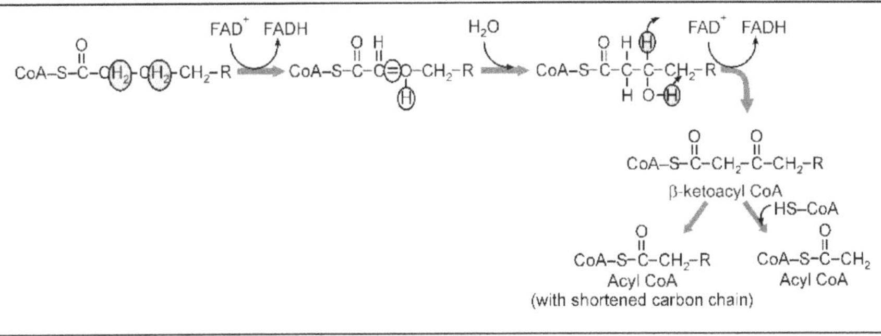

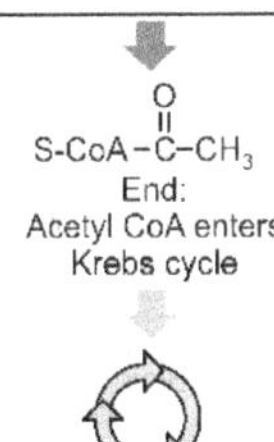

Fig. 8.4 The β-oxidation of fatty acids.

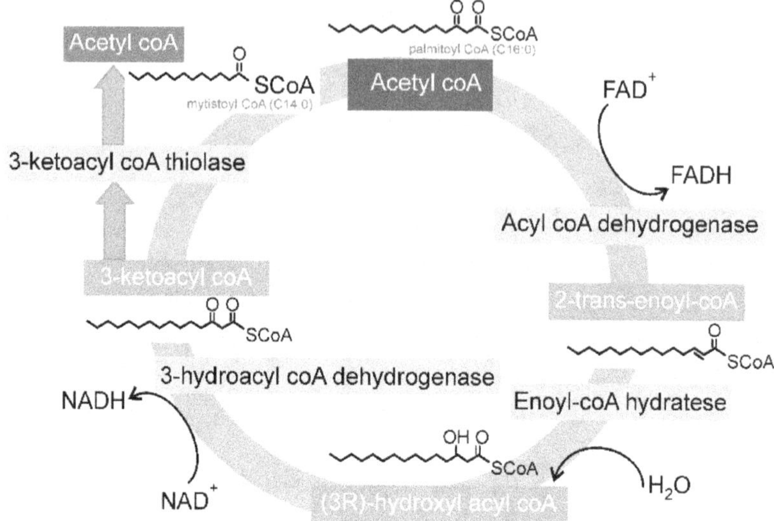

Fig. 8.5 The β-oxidation of palmitic acid.

Ketone Bodies

Ketone bodies include compounds specially acetone, acetoacetate and β-hydroxybutyrate or 3-hydroxybutyrate) **Fig. 8.6**. The compounds acetone and acetoacetate possess a keto (C=O) group and are true ketones whereas β-hydroxybutyrate lacks keto group. The ketone bodies are highly soluble in water and yields energy. The acetone, compound cannot be metabolized and is an exception.

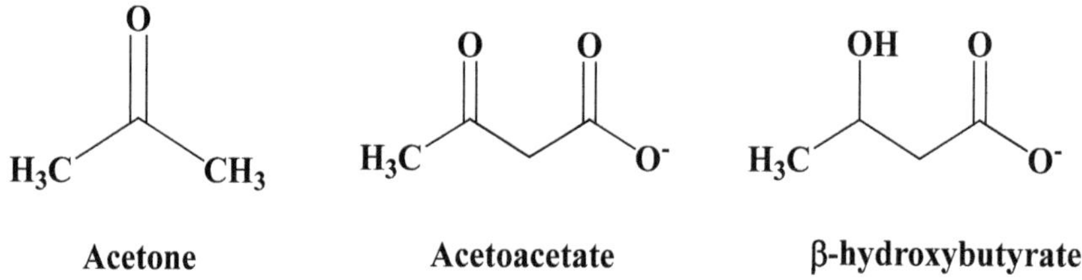

Fig. 8.6 Chemical Structures of ketone bodies.

Ketogenesis

The ketone bodies are synthesized in the liver whereas enzymes responsible. The enzymes responsible for ketone body generation are present in the mitochondrial matrix. The precursors for ketogenesis are acetyl CoA (final product of β-oxidation of fatty acids) and pyruvate or amino acids. is the precursor for ketone bodies. The key steps involved in ketogenesis are:

1. In the first step, the thiolase enzyme catalyses acetyl CoA (2moles) give acetoacetyl CoA.

2. Further, in presence of HMG CoA synthase enzyme acetoacetyl CoA reacts with acetyl CoA to form β-hydroxy-β-methyl glutaryl CoA (HMG CoA).

3. In this step, HMG CoA lyase enzyme separates HMG CoA to form acetoacetate and acetyl CoA.

4. Further, the decarboxylation of acetoacetate leads to the formation of acetone.

5. Whereas the reduction of acetoacetate in presence of enzyme dehydrogenase forms β-hydroxybutyrate.

The steps involved in ketogenesis are shown in **Fig. 8.7.**

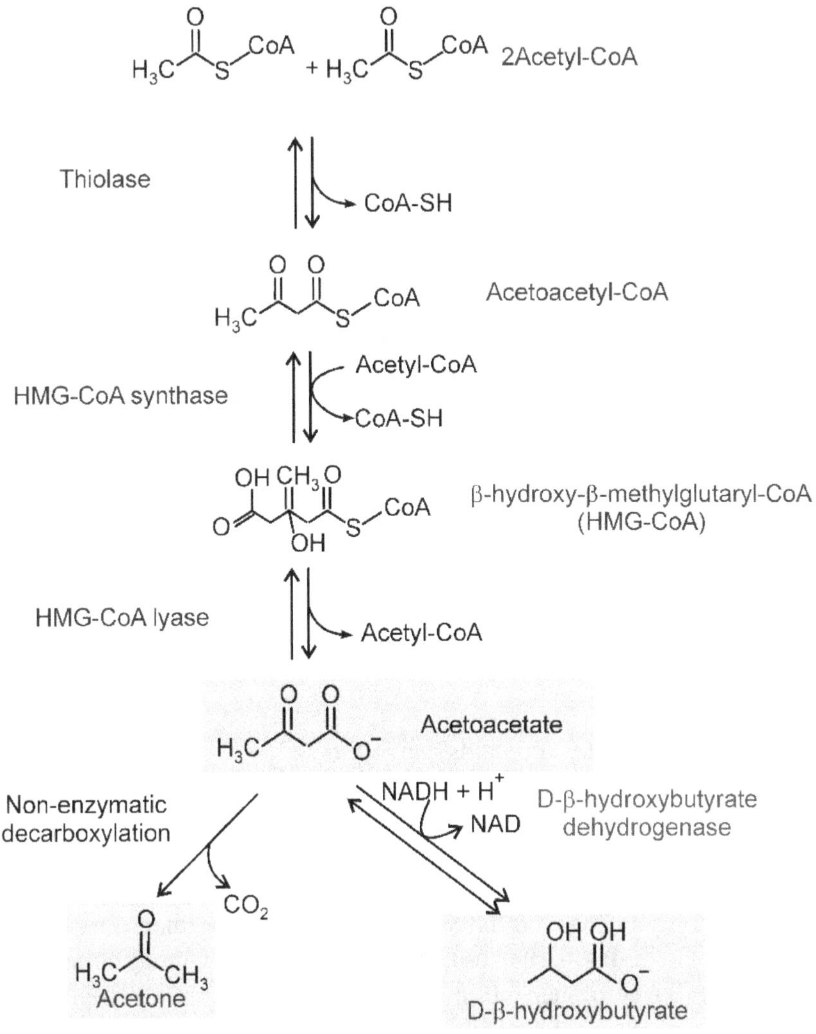

Fig. 8.7 The ketogenesis pathway or generation of ketone bodies.

Ketolysis

The catabolism of ketone bodies inside body is known as ketolysis. This process is just opposite to ketogenesis (formation of ketone bodies).

Salient features of ketolysis pathway:

- Ketolysis process is major pathway for energy supply and ATP generation apart from β-oxidation.

- The primary site for ketogenesis is liver whereas the ketolysis process operates in non-living cells or peripheral tissues like skeletal muscle, heart and brain region.

- The main enzyme responsible for ketolysis is Succinyl-CoA:3-ketoacid CoA transferase (SCOT) which is found in the mitochondria of all mammalian cells except other than hepatocytes.

- Ketone bodies are main source of fuel at the time of long starvation, serving the brain and central nervous system parts.

Diseases Related to Abnormal Metabolism of Lipids

Ketoacidosis

It is defined as elevation in the concentration of strong acidic ketone bodies i.e., acetoacetate and β-hydroxybutyrate in blood. Generally, rise in strong acid in blood is termed as acidosis and ketoacidosis is the term for ketone bodies which are acidic in nature and their level increases in the blood. The pKa value of carboxyl group is 4. So, the ketone bodies get broken down in the blood and liberates H^+ and decreases pH. Severe form of ketoacidosis is "diabetic ketoacidosis" - a critical situation which if not treated timely may lead to coma or death conditions. Ketosis due to starvation is not usually accompanied by ketoacidosis. The treatment for ketoacidosis is to maintain water and electrolyte balance. Insulin injection helps in the utilization of glucose by through tissues and blockage of ketogenesis pathway.

Fatty liver

Human liver generally contains approximately 5% of fats or more specifically phospholipids. As liver is not an organ for fat storage just like adipose tissue. So, fatty liver can be defined as a condition in which lipids specifically triacylglycerols get enormously deposited in cytoplasm of hepatic cells other than kupffer cells of liver. This leads to change in metabolic activity of liver. In fatty liver condition, liver undergoes cirrhosis and changes in fibrous tissue formation. Fatty liver is caused either due to elevated triacylglycerol generation or change in production of lipoproteins in the body.

Hypercholesterolemia

It is defined as rise in cholesterol level in blood plasma i.e., more than 200mg/dL. Increased cholesterol level is seen in various disorders like atherosclerosis, coronary heart disease (CHD), diabetes mellitus, hypothyroidism or myxoedema, obstructive jaundice and nephrotic syndrome etc. The cholesterol found in LDL (low-density lipoproteins) is generally considered bad due its high concentration and association with atherosclerosis and related conditions. This may be regarded as "lethally dangerous lipoprotein" and sits sub form sd LDL i.e, small dens LDL is designated as "most dangerous fraction" of LDL which is responsible for CHD. Whereas HDL or high-density lipoprotein is regarded as "good cholesterol" or highly desirable lipoprotein due its counter action effect towards atherogenesis.

Biological Oxidation

Biological oxidation is defined as sequence of oxidation reduction conversions of biomolecules in living organisms. The biological oxidation is an enzyme catalysed process which works with the union of coenzymes and electron carrier proteins. There is conversion of energy rich molecule to low energy compound with release of heat energy which further gets converted to ATP in the form of chemical energy. The term "bioenergetics" refers to energy concerned with construction and destruction of chemical bonds in the biomolecules.

Electron Transport Chain (ETC)

The transmission of electrons through substrate towards molecular oxygen with the help of a chain of electron carriers is known as electron transport chain (ETC) or respiratory chain. The biomolecules like carbohydrates (glucose), lipids (fatty acids) and proteins (amino acids) which are rich in energy gets oxidised to CO_2 and H_2O through series of metabolic reactions. This causes conversion of reducing equivalents generated through metabolic reactions to get transferred to coenzymes NAD^+ and FAD. These Coenzymes then further get converted to their reduced form i.e., NADH and $FADH_2$ which later get used in ETC with the release of water molecule from half molecule of oxygen and ATP from ADP and inorganic phosphate (Pi).

Site of ETC

The site for ETC assembly is inner membrane(cristae) of mitochondrion. The mitochondrion is also known as "storage power house of cell" because it is the major site for most of the metabolic oxidative reactions which produce reduced coenzymes i.e., NADH and $FADH_2$. These reduced coenzymes are used in ETC to generate energy in the form of ATP. The components and reactions of ETC is shown in **Fig. 8.8.**

Components and reactions of ETC

Electron transport chain works with the involvement of five components or complexes (Complex I, II, III, IV &V). The complex I-IV act as electron carriers whereas complex V is involved in ATP synthesis. Apart from these various mobile electron carriers like oxygen, NADH, Coenzyme Q, and cytochrome C etc. work as electron transporters in the ETC. Finally, all complexes(I-IV) and mobile electron carriers couples with oxygen to generate water molecule. So, mitochondrion uses larger fraction of oxygen for the proper functioning of ETC. Each complex is briefly discussed here:

I. Nicotinamide nucleotides

Complex I consist of niacin vitamin derivative coenzymes NAD^+ and $NADP^+$. Out of these two coenzymes NAD^+ effectively participates in ETC. The dehydrogenases enzymes reduce NAD^+ to $NADH + H^+$ with the liberation of two hydrogen atoms out of AH_2 substrate. Whereas NADPH is used in anabolic reactions like fatty acid and cholesterol biosynthesis. The enzyme involved in this complex is NADH coQ reductase.

II. Flavoproteins

The coenzyme FMN (flavin mononucleotide) or riboflavin-5'-phosphate functions as prosthetic group in the enzyme NADH coenzyme Q reductase or NADH dehydrogenase. The FMN gets converted to $FMNH_2$ by gaining a proton and two electrons. The complex enzyme NADH dehydrogenase is involved in catalysis of non-heme iron or sulfur iron proteins. Another enzyme associated with complex II is succinate coenzyme Q reductase or succinate dehydrogenase which exists in inner part of mitochondrion. The FAD (flavin adenine dinucleotide) functions as coenzyme in this flavoprotein and forms fumarate and $FADH_2$ by the gain of two hydrogen atoms through succinate.

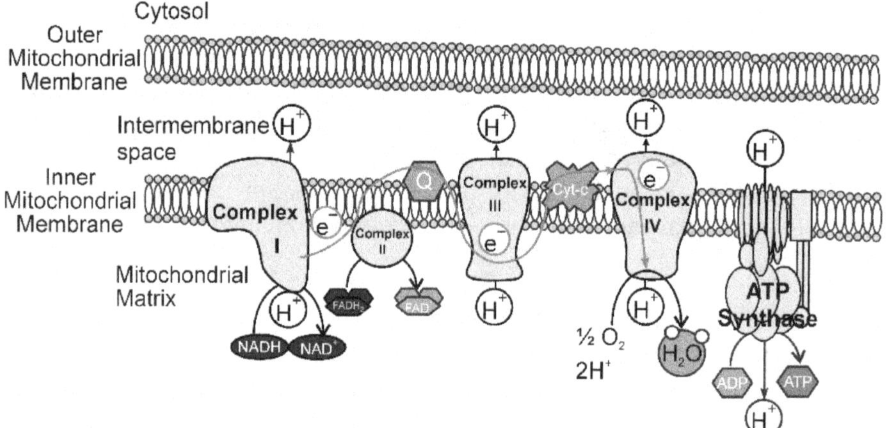

Fig. 8.8 The electron transport chain.

III. Iron-sulfur proteins (FeS)

The FeS proteins are present in complex IV either as reduced form i.e., Fe^{2+} or in oxidised form i.e., Fe^{3+}. These proteins are involved in transportation of electrons through FMN towards coenzyme Q and in between cytochromes (cytochrome b and c_1).

IV. Coenzyme Q (Ubiquinone)

Coenzyme Q or ubiquinone is derived from quinone compound with side as isoprenoid units. The coenzyme Q_{10} or CoQ_{10} consists of ten isoprenoid units. It is involved in lipophilic electron transport. It gains electrons through $FMNH_2$ generated inside ETC with the help of $FADH_2$ or NADH dehydrogenase enzyme (generated outside ETC).

V. Cytochromes

These are conjugate proteins having heme group i.e., iron trapped inside porphyrin ring. The iron associate with these proteins is actively involved in transportation of electrons inside ETC by the interconversion from oxidised state (Fe^{3+}) to reduced state (Fe^{2+}). The cytochrome enzymes are named as "a, b, c" according to the type of iron present but later cytochromes c_1, b_1, b_2, a_3 also came in existence. The flow of electrons inside ETC from coenzyme Q towards cytochromes is in the order b, c_1, c, a and finally through a_3. The reversible oxidation-reduction of heme or iron present inside cytochrome proteins makes them perfect electron transporter of electrons in ETC.

Inhibitors of ETC

The ETC inhibitors are responsible for blocking the electron transport chain by blocking the components and site of ETC occurrence. The inhibitors bind to following three main sites in ETC:

1. **NADH and Coenzyme Q:** This site is inhibited by rotenone (fish poison), Amytal (a barbiturate drug), and piercidin A (an antibiotic).

2. **Between cytochrome b and c_1:** This site is inhibited by antimycin A (an antibiotic) and BAL or British antilewisite (an antidote used for war gas poisoning).

3. **Cytochrome oxidase inhibitors:** These include hydrogen sulphide, cyanide, carbon monoxide, and azide.

Oxidative Phosphorylation

Simply oxidation linked with phosphorylation is known as oxidative phosphorylation. It is defined as process of ATP generation through ADP (adenosine diphosphate) and Pi (inorganic phosphate) when transfer of electrons through electron carriers takes place from NADH or $FADH_2$ towards oxygen in ETC. The P:O ratio indicates the total of inorganic phosphates used for ATP synthesis for each oxygen atom utilized during oxidative phosphorylation.

Site of Oxidative Phosphorylation

The location of oxidative phosphorylation is complex V which is present inside the inner membrane(cristae) of mitochondria. However, the oxidative phosphorylation occurs at three sites in electron transport chain (ETC) as:

(a) $FMNH_2$ oxidation through coenzyme Q

(b) Cytochrome b oxidation through cytochrome c_1

(c) Cytochrome oxidase enzyme reaction

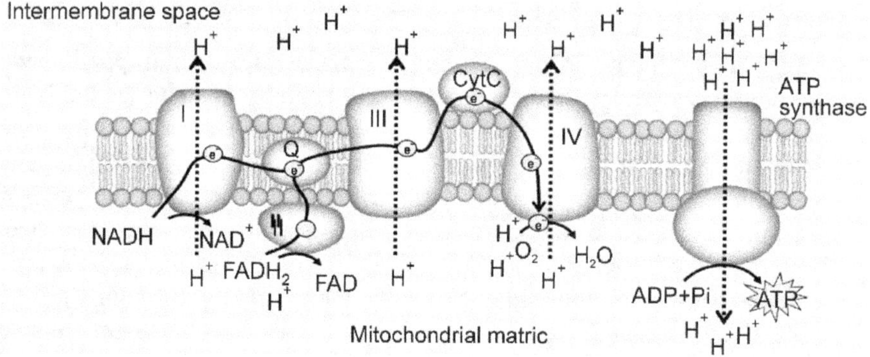

Fig. 8.9 The oxidative phosphorylation.

Mechanism of Oxidative Phosphorylation

Many hypotheses have been reported to explain the oxidative phosphorylation process. The most important of them are chemical coupling hypothesis and chemiosmotic theory.

1. **Chemical coupling hypothesis**

   This hypothesis was given by Edward Slater in 1953. This hypothesis states that during electron transport chain operation a sequence of high energy phosphorylated intermediates are synthesized first which are then further used for the generation of ATP. All these reactions occur similarly to substrate level phosphorylation which takes place in citric acid cycle or glycolysis. But this hypothesis does not have any experimental confirmation.

2. **Chemiosmotic theory**

   This hypothesis was given by the scientist Peter Mitchell in 1961 and was awarded noble prize in 1978. This hypothesis is widely accepted and explains that how electrons get transported in ETC and are used to generate ATP through ADP and inorganic phosphate. The basic principles behind this theory are: -

(a) Proton pumping through electron carrier proteins

(b) Development of Electrochemical potential

   (i) Membrane potential

   (ii) Chemical potential or proton gradient

(c) Transportation of electron flow finally back to matrix by ATPase enzyme.

The inner membrane of mitochondria is impermeable towards H^+ and OH^- ions. The electron transportation is concerned with the translocation of H^+ ions towards the inner membrane of mitochondria. The translocation of H^+ is intended towards intermembrane space from the matrix. This results in generation of electrochemical or proton gradient.

Uncouplers

These are the compounds which delink or uncouple the electron transport chain process from the oxidative phosphorylation resulting in the permeability of H^+ ions towards mitochondrial inner membrane and inhibits ATP synthesis. The uncouplers carry out oxidation of substrates through NADH or $FADH_2$ at high speed without ATP generation. The examples of uncouplers include 2,4-dinitrophenol (DNP), dinitrocresol, phenylhydrazone (FCCP), trifluorocarbonylcyanide, pentachlorophenol, and aspirin (at high doses). These all uncouplers may be called as ionophores or proton ionophores as these enhance permeability of ions through biological membrane. The antibiotics like nigercin, valinomycin, and gramicidin A also work as K^+ ion ionophores.

The uncoupling phenomenon finds its significance in animals adapted to cold or hibernating animals and hairless animals regarding body temperature maintenance. These animals possess special type of fat tissues called brown adipose tissue (upper back and neck parts of body). The mitochondria present inside the brown tissue possess high quantity of electron carriers which are specialized to perform oxidation uncoupled phosphorylation. This process results in release of heat when fat gets oxidized in brown adipose tissues and animals don't become obese. The consumption of excessive calories by these animals gets burn and released in the form of heat and result is no deposition of fat in their bodies.

The thermogenin acts as physiological uncoupling protein which blocks ATP synthesis by the inhibition of oxidative phosphorylation coupled with ETC. Other uncouplers include oligomycin and atractyloside etc.

Metabolism of Amino Acids (Proteins)

Protein are nitrogen containing complex macromolecules which upon breakdown or proteolysis give single L-α-amino acids. The sum of all the amino acids present inside a human body is known amino acid pool of the body. Generally, on an average an adult's body contain 100g of free amino acids. Therefore, protein metabolism can be precisely studied as amino acid metabolism.

Transamination

When amino group(-NH$_2$) of α-amino acid gets exchanged with oxo group of a keto acid or 2-oxo acid from, this phenomenon is known transamination. This process comprises of amino acids, keto acids and enzymes transaminases or aminotransferases. There is involvement of coenzyme pyridoxal phosphate or PLP (vitamin B6 derived coenzyme) by the enzyme transaminases. Transamination helps in reorganization of amino acids and generation of non-essential amino acids through the catabolism or anabolism phenomenon. Examples of transamination include enzymes aspartate aminotransferase (AST) and alanine aminotransferase (ALT) which are used in diagnosis of liver related diseases.

Deamination

When amino group gets removed from an amino acid in the form of ammonia (NH$_3$) then this phenomenon is known deamination. The ammonia liberated here undergoes urea cycle to form urea. The remaining carbon skeleton after the removal of ammonia, gets converted to keto acids. It is of two types: oxidative and non-oxidative deamination.

(a) Oxidative deamination: It is defined as the deamination or amino group removal linked with oxidation process. This phenomenon plays key role in urea synthesis by supplying NH$_3$.

(b) Non-oxidative deamination: It is oxidation free deamination generally followed by some amino acids like serine, homoserine, hydroxyamino acids, cysteine, and histidine etc.

Urea Cycle

Urea cycle was the first metabolic pathway that was described by scientists Hans Krebs and Kurt Henseleit in 1932. Therefore, this pathway is also called as Krebs-Henseleit cycle. The ammonia generated from metabolism of amino acids is highly toxic to the body. To reduce its toxicity, it gets transformed to urea and gets detoxified through urea cycle. The final or end product of protein or amino acid metabolism is urea which further gets excreted out of the body through urine. The steps involved in urea cycle are outlined in the **Fig. 8.10**.

Site of urea cycle

The urea cycle occurs in liver whereas urea gets excreted out of the body through kidneys. The synthesis of urea follows five steps. The enzymes responsible for first two steps are located in mitochondria whereas enzymes for step three to five are present in the cytosol of liver cells.

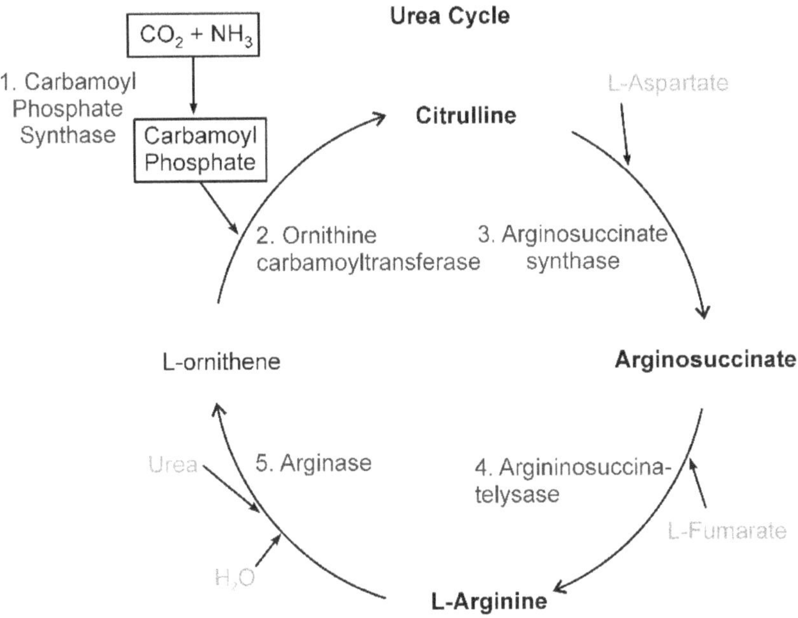

Fig. 8.10 The urea cycle.

Reactions of Urea Cycle

Step 1. Carbamoyl phosphate synthesis: The urea cycle starts with the condensation reaction of carbon dioxide and ammonia in presence of enzyme carbamoyl phosphate synthase-I (CPS-I) which is situated inside the mitochondria of liver cells. N-acetyl glutamate (NAG) is required by CPS-I for its catalytic activity. This step utilises two ATP to form two ADP's and an inorganic phosphate. This reaction is a rate limiting step and irreversible in nature.

Step 2. Generation of citrulline: The main first component of the urea cycle citrulline gets synthesized from the carbamoyl phosphate and ornithine (present in cytosol) in presence of enzyme ornithine transcarbamoylase. This step occurs in mitochondria.

Step 3. Arginosuccinate formation: In this step, citrulline gets converted to arginosuccinate in presence of aspartate and an enzyme arginosuccinate synthase. This step utilises ATP which gets cleaved to AMP and pyrophosphate (PPi). The pyrophosphate further gets converted to inorganic phosphate (Pi).

Step 4. Breakdown of arginosuccinate: The arginosuccinate gets broken down into fumarate and arginine in presence of enzyme arginosuccinase. The arginine formed in this step acts as precursor for urea generation. Whereas, fumarate gets utilized in gluconeogenesis and Krebs cycle etc.

Step 5. Generation of urea: The arginine formed in the step 4 gets further cleaved to ornithine and final product urea in presence of enzyme arginase. The ornithine formed is further reutilized in the urea cycle. The urea generated in this step gets further transported to kidney where it gets excreted out in urine. The arginase enzyme used in this step is only present in liver cells whereas other four enzymes are also found in other tissues. This is the reason that only liver can synthesize urea in the body.

Energetics of Urea cycle

Urea cycle utilizes a total of four ATP molecules. Two ATP are used in the generation of carbamoyl phosphate. Whereas, one ATP utilized during arginosuccinate formation. This ATP get broken down to AMP and PPi which is equivalent to two ATP.

Decarboxylation

It is defined as elimination of carbon dioxide (CO_2) from amino acids through the decarboxylases enzymes with generation of amines. The amines formed further act as hormones or neurotransmitters with some physiological action. The decarboxylases enzyme requires a coenzyme pyridoxal-phospahte for its function. The decarboxylation is important as it helps in generation of physiological active compounds hormones (epinephrine, melatonin, thyroxine etc.) and neurotransmitters (serotonin, dopamine, GABA etc.). The decarboxylation also contributes during catabolism or degradation of amino acids or protein with the generation of diamines. For example, ornithine and lysine get degraded to their diamine compounds putrescine and cadaverine respectively.

Disorders of Ammonia Metabolism

Ammonia metabolism disorders include hyperammonaemia I &II caused due to defective enzymes carbamoyl phosphate synthase I and ornithine transcarbamoylase respectively. Other disorders are citrullinemia, arginosuccinic aciduria, and hyperaginimia cause by defective enzymes arginosuccinate synthase, arginosuccinase, and arginase respectively. All these ammonia disorders finally cause hyperammonemia or excessive accumulation of ammonia in the blood which can cause severe toxicity. Symptoms include mental retardation, vomiting, lethargy, and irritation etc.

Diseases Related to Abnormal Metabolism of Amino Acids

The abnormal metabolism amino acid leads to various diseases like phenylketonuria, alkaptonuria, and maple syrup urine disease (MSUD) etc.

Phenylketonuria

This disorder is commonly called as PKU is an inherited disease which elevates level of phenylalanine in the body. Change in phenylalanine hydroxylase (PAH) gene leads to phenylketonuria disease. This gene is responsible for metabolism or lysis of phenylalanine. This disease is caused due to the lack of enzyme phenylalanine hydroxylase which is a hepatic enzyme. Symptoms of this disease include mental retardation, frequent seizures, and hypopigmentation (blue eyes and lightening of skin and hairs) etc. This disease can be treated by maintaining the normal concentration of phenylalanine in the blood plasma. This can be done by consuming the food items low in phenylalanine content.

Alkaptonuria

Alkaptonuria also known as black urine disease is a rare disease that blocks break down of tyrosine and phenylalanine amino acids. This results in formation of homogentisic acid inside the body. This is an inherited disorder and can change colour of urine and skin to black. The enzyme homogentisate oxidase (involved in tyrosine metabolism) oxidises homogentisate to benzoquinone acetate which further encounters polymerization reaction to form a pigment called 'alkapton'. This alkapton get deposited in the connective tissues, nose, ear and bones etc. leading to a skin condition called 'ochronosis'. This disease does not require any special treatment but consumption of food with low amount of phenylalanine is recommended.

Jaundice (Icterus)

Jaundice (French word Jaune-yellow) is a disease characterised by symptoms like yellowish discoloration of mucous membrane and white part of eyes. Jaundice is caused due to the overproduction of a bile pigment 'bilirubin" also known as hyperbilirubinemia and deposition of bile pigments. Bilirubin is a yellowish-orange bile pigment generated due to the lysis of red blood cells and is secreted by the liver and in the bone marrow cells. Jaundice is also caused due to an inherited enzyme deficiency called glucose-6-phosphate dehydrogenase(G6PD). Clinically jaundice can be detected by the determination of elevated plasma bilirubin concentration i.e.,

50μmol/L or 3mg/dL. The chronic jaundice may lead to severe cause of diseases like tumours, gallstones and hepatitis etc. There are three types of jaundice;

(a) Hemolytic jaundice-caused due to increased haemolysis (RBC breakdown).

(b) Hepatic jaundice-caused due to dysfunction of liver or defect in parenchymal cells.

(c) Obstructive jaundice-caused due to blockage in the bile duct

> **Chapter 9**

Minerals

Minerals are typically compounds that meet five characteristics. They have a well-organized internal structure and are 1) naturally occurring, 2) inorganic, 3) solid, 4) chemically defined, and 5) inorganic. Minerals play an important role in our everyday lives and constitute the bulk of the earth's mass. They are characterised as naturally occurring crystalline substances. Similar to vitamins, minerals contribute to the growth, development, and maintenance of the body. Oxygen, silicon, copper, iron, calcium, sodium, potassium, and magnesium make up approximately 99 percent of the Earth's crust's minerals. The minerals quartz, feldspar, bauxite, cobalt, talc, and pyrite are prevalent. Some minerals have a contrasting stripe of colour on their bodies. Minerals are utilised by the body for a range of functions, including bone production and nerve impulse transmission. A nutritionist uses the term mineral to refer to the numerous inorganic components organisms need to grow, repair tissue, metabolise, and carry out other physiological tasks. Numerous minerals, including iron, calcium, copper, sulphur, phosphorus, and magnesium, are needed for human health. Some minerals are also necessary for hormone synthesis and maintaining a normal heartbeat. Calcium is the most prevalent mineral in the human body, comprising 1.5 to 2 percent of total body mass. The majority of the approximately 1,200 g of calcium in an adult's body is found in their bones.

The following is a list of potential causes of mineral insufficiency in the body:

- A lack of essential minerals in the diet or via supplements is one of the most prevalent causes of mineral deficit.

- There are several types of diets that may result in this deficiency. A poor diet heavy in junk food or devoid of fruits and vegetables may be contributing causes; a very low-calorie diet may be the cause. This includes those on a weight-loss programme or with an eating disorder. It is also conceivable that elderly individuals with poor appetites do not consume enough calories or nutrients. Dietary restrictions can also induce mineral deficits. Mineral deficiency can arise among vegetarians, vegans, and people with food allergies or lactose intolerance who do not control their diet adequately.

- Mineral deficiencies can be caused by issues with food digestion or nutrition absorption. These disorders may be caused by a variety of reasons, such as liver, gallbladder, intestinal, pancreatic, and renal diseases; surgery to the digestive tract; and persistent alcoholism.

- An increased need for certain minerals may also result in mineral deficiency. This need may occur during pregnancy, heavy menstruation, or menopause.

Uses of Some Minerals in the Body

Iron: Iron performs several essential functions in the body. It serves as a transporter of oxygen from the lungs to the tissues via haemoglobin in red blood cells, as a medium for electron transport inside cells, and as a component of essential enzyme systems in several organs. Iron's physiology has been extensively studied. Haemoglobin, a molecule composed of four units, each of which consists of one haem group and one protein chain, holds the bulk of the body's iron. The structure of haemoglobin permits it to be fully loaded with oxygen in the lungs and partially unloaded in the tissues (for example, in the muscles). Myoglobin is an iron-containing oxygen storage protein found in muscles. Its structure is similar to that of haemoglobin, but it contains just one haem unit and one globin chain. One haem group and one globin protein chain are also present in cytochromes, a kind of iron-containing enzymes. Iron-containing enzymes are essential for the manufacture of steroid hormones and bile acids, as well as the detoxification of foreign substances in the liver and signal control in particular neurotransmitter systems, such as the dopamine and serotonin systems in the brain (e.g. cytochrome P450). Iron is stored reversibly in the liver as ferritin and haemosiderin, and it is transported across body compartments via the transferrin protein. It facilitates oxygen supply to muscles. Iron is necessary for cell growth, development, and proper functioning of the body. Iron contributes to the formation of hormones and connective tissue in the body. Approximately 99 percent of the body's calcium is kept in bones, while the remaining 1 percent is found in blood, muscle, and other tissues. The body attempts to maintain a steady calcium content in the blood and tissues in order to carry out these vital daily operations. When calcium levels in the blood get too low, parathyroid hormone (PTH) instructs the bones to release calcium into the circulation. This hormone may also activate vitamin D, allowing for enhanced intestinal calcium absorption. Additionally, PTH orders the kidneys to excrete less calcium into the urine. When the body has sufficient calcium, a hormone known as calcitonin reduces blood calcium levels by blocking calcium from being released from the bones and instructing the kidneys to flush more of it through urine. Calcium is acquired by the body in two ways. The first is to eat calcium-rich meals or supplements; the second is to remove calcium from the body. If you do not eat enough calcium-rich foods, your body will remove calcium from your bones. In principle, calcium "borrowed" from the bones should be returned at a later time. This is not always the case, nor is it always easy to achieve by taking additional calcium. Calcium is present in several multivitamin-mineral supplements, calcium supplements, and supplements including calcium and other minerals such as vitamin D. Other calcium forms included in dietary supplements and fortified foods include calcium sulphate, calcium ascorbate, calcium microcrystalline hydroxyapatite, calcium gluconate, calcium lactate, and calcium phosphate.

Sodium: Sodium is a second important mineral. Sodium facilitates muscle contraction, transmits nerve signals, and maintains fluid equilibrium in the body. The most prevalent source of sodium in the diet is table salt. In contrast, salt should be eaten in moderation. Sodium is essential to the survival of all animals and certain plants. Sodium is the predominant cation in extracellular fluid (ECF), contributing greatly to ECF osmotic pressure and compartment capacity. When ECF compartment water is lost, the salt content rises, resulting in hypernatremia. In a condition known as ECF hypovolemia, the ECF compartment becomes smaller due to the isotonic loss of water and salt. Living human cells utilise the sodium-potassium pump to pump three sodium ions out of the cell in exchange for two potassium ions; when comparing ion concentrations within and outside the cell membrane, potassium is around 40:1 and sodium is approximately 1:10. Sodium plays a crucial part in the transmission of nerve impulses, also known as action potentials, when the electrical charge across the cell membrane is dissipated in nerve cells. The renin–angiotensin system is responsible for regulating the body's fluid and sodium levels. Renin is created when blood pressure and salt levels decrease in the kidney, which subsequently produces aldosterone and angiotensin, which promote sodium reabsorption. As sodium concentration increases, renin synthesis decreases, and sodium concentration returns to normal. The sodium ion (Na^+) is vital for neuronal activation and osmoregulation between cells and extracellular fluid. Sodium/potassium channels and Na^+/K^+-ATPase, an active transporter that pumps ions against the gradient, are responsible for this in all organisms. Sodium is the most prevalent metal ion in extracellular fluid. Hyponatremia and hypernatremia refer to unusually low or high sodium levels in the blood of humans. These issues may be caused by genetic causes, ageing, or persistent vomiting or diarrhoea.

Potassium: Potassium is a necessary mineral for the proper operation of your cells, neurons, and muscles. It is a systemic electrolyte that aids in the regulation of ATP by sodium. It helps regulate blood pressure, heart rhythm, and the water content of cells. The vast majority of individuals obtain all of their potassium through meals and beverages. It is also available as a dietary supplement. Potassium is an essential element for all of the body's tissues. It is frequently referred to as an electrolyte because it contains a small electrical charge that activates a variety of cellular and neuronal functions. Its principal purpose in the body is to aid in maintaining the correct fluid levels within our cells. In contrast, sodium maintains proper fluid levels outside of cells. Potassium also promotes muscular contraction and good blood pressure. Potassium is necessary for fluid homeostasis, muscular contraction, and nerve signal transmission. It improves mental health and reduces the chance of stroke. Low potassium levels cause, among other things, irregular heartbeats, oedema (swelling), and brain damage. Bananas, sweet potatoes, avocados, beets, and dates are rich in potassium. The kidneys maintain appropriate potassium levels in the blood by eliminating excess potassium through urine. Additionally, potassium is lost via the intestines and perspiration. Hypokalemia can be induced by any condition that results in significant fluid loss, such as vomiting, diarrhoea, or some medications, such as diuretics. Hypokalemia is more prevalent in hospitalised patients who are taking medications that increase potassium excretion. Inflammatory bowel diseases (Crohn's disease, ulcerative colitis) can also cause nutritional loss and diarrhoea. Potassium deficiency is unusual since potassium is present in so many foods; nonetheless, an inadequate intake coupled with excessive sweating, diuretic usage, laxative misuse, or severe nausea and vomiting can rapidly result in hypokalemia. As the kidneys require magnesium to reabsorb potassium and maintain normal cell levels, magnesium deficiency is another reason.

Chlorine: Together with sodium, chloride maintains the body's fluid equilibrium. It promotes digestion by producing hydrochloric acid (stomach acid) and preserving the body's electrical neutrality. It is necessary for both the production of hydrochloric acid in the stomach and the operation of the cellular pump. The chloride anion is an essential ingredient for metabolism. Electrolyte disorders are characterised by either low or excessive blood chloride concentrations. In the absence of further conditions, hypochloraemia (a lack of chloride in the blood) is unusual. It is occasionally associated to hypoventilation. It has been connected with chronic respiratory acidosis. Typically, hyperchloremia (excess chloride in the blood) is asymptomatic. When symptoms do manifest, they are frequently misdiagnosed as hypernatremia (having too much sodium). Cerebral dehydration is precipitated by a reduction in blood chloride; symptoms are typically precipitated by rapid rehydration, which induces cerebral oedema. Hyperchloremia can hinder the transportation of oxygen. After ingestion, chlorine is readily absorbed, but it is also rapidly eliminated via perspiration, renal excretion, and intestinal evacuation. When heavy perspiration diminishes the body's fluid level during hot weather, the body's chlorine stores are rapidly depleted. Also, during periods of severe vomiting and diarrhoea, as well as situations that produce severe alkalosis, or a build-up of base or loss of acid in the body, the body's stored chlorides may drop to dangerously low levels. **Table 9.1** illustrates the daily mineral requirement, their sources and deficiency diseases.

Table 9.1 Mineral requirement and their associated diseases.

Mineral	Daily requirement Male/ Female (mg)	Source	Deficiency diseases
Iron	8/18	Iron is abundant in green leafy vegetables, dark chocolates, nuts and meats such as beef, poultry, and pork.	Anemia (short of breath, tiredness)
Calcium	1000	Dairy products, eggs, tinned fish with bones (salmon, sardines), green leafy vegetables, nuts, seeds, tofu, thyme, oregano, dill, cinnamon, thyme, ore, cashews, dates, broccoli, parsley, and greens.	Hypocalcaemia, osteoporosis, dental problems, depression, severe premenstrual syndrome (PMS)
Sodium	1000	Salt (sodium chloride, the primary source), plant foods, milk, and spinach are all good sources of sodium chloride.	Hyponatremia
Potassium	4700	Potassium is abundant in bananas, sweet potatoes, avocados, beets, and dates, as well as tomatoes, potatoes, beans, lentils, dairy products, shellfish, bananas, prunes, carrots, oranges, pinach, and broccoli, water made from coconuts, greens from beets, almonds and cashews, cantaloupe, chicken and Salmon	Hypokalemia
Chlorine	2300	Table salt, tomatoes, celery, lettuce, meat, eggs and milk are major sources of chlorine.	Hypochloremia

> **Chapter 10**

Water and Electrolytes

Around 60 to 70 percent of the human body's weight is comprised of water, making it the most plentiful component. It is essential to life, and humans cannot survive more than a few days without it. Water serves as a component of cells and bodily fluids, as well as a medium for chemical reactions, a solvent, and a reactant. Additionally, it delivers nutrients and facilitates in the elimination of waste through urine. Sweat evaporation is vital for the control of body temperature. To maintain this proportion of water in humans, water as a nutritional source is crucial. Infants contain more water than adults do. Water is only second in significance to oxygen to the human organism. It is possible to survive without food for longer than without water. Water is a tasteless, calorie-free combination of hydrogen and oxygen that is essential for the survival of virtually all body cells. Other uses of water include the protection of the spinal cord and other delicate tissues, the elimination of waste through urine, perspiration, and bowel movements, the lubrication and cushioning of joints, and the regulation of body temperature.

In water, compounds dissolve as positively and negatively charged ions. Electrolytes is the term for these substances. Sodium, potassium, and chloride are the most prevalent electrolytes inside the human body. Therefore, water is capable of dissolving the majority of substances, allowing minerals and other molecules to participate in biological activities within the body. Water is the most essential component of the human body; it is present in every organ, as well as between and between cells. The overall quantity of salt in the body determines the body's total water content. The kidneys manage the body's sodium and water levels. The average water content of various bodily parts is shown in the following **Table 10.1**.

Table 10.1 The average water content in various body parts.

Body part	Water percentage
Brain	82-85%
Heart	75-78%
Kidneys	82-85%

Table 10.1 *Contd...*

Body part	Water percentage
Skin	72-75%
Liver	70-73%
Bones	17-25%
Teeth	8-10%

Cell membranes allow water to flow in and out of body cells.

(a) Intracellular fluids: It is neither a continuous phase, nor is it a homogeneous phase; rather, it is the total amount of fluid that is contained inside all of the cells in the body. The amount of water present as well as the ionic make-up of a cell's cytoplasm, nucleus, mitochondria, and microsomes may vary greatly depending on the kind of cell. This is due to the fact that a cell has a large number of anatomic sub-divisions. This intracellular fluid accounts for thirty to forty percent of the body's entire mass and contains around fifty-five percent of the body's total water.

(b) Extracellular fluids: Approximately one-third of the total fluid in the body is made up of fluid that is found outside of cells. This category of fluid includes intravascular and interstitial fluids. Extracellular fluids include interstitial fluid, which is water found between cells, intravascular fluid, which is water found in the blood stream and lymph, and lymph fluid. It is believed that water makes up 55% of the space found inside of cells as well as the remaining 45% of the space found outside of cells. The tissue cells and the bloodstream are connected by the interstitial fluid, which acts as a conduit. The extracellular fluid phase is subdivided into the following groups when examined further:

1. 2.5 percent transcellular water.

2. Water content of dense connective tissue and cartilage is 7.5 percent.

3. 7.5 percent of plasma water is contained within the circulatory system.

4. Lymph and interstitial fluid- 20 percent.

5. Bone water that is inaccessible- 7.5 percent.

Edelman and collaborators (1952) coined the term "transcellular" to describe extracellular fluid that has been separated from other extracellular fluid by an epithelial membrane. The following substances are found in this transcellular fluid illustrated in **Fig. 10.1**.

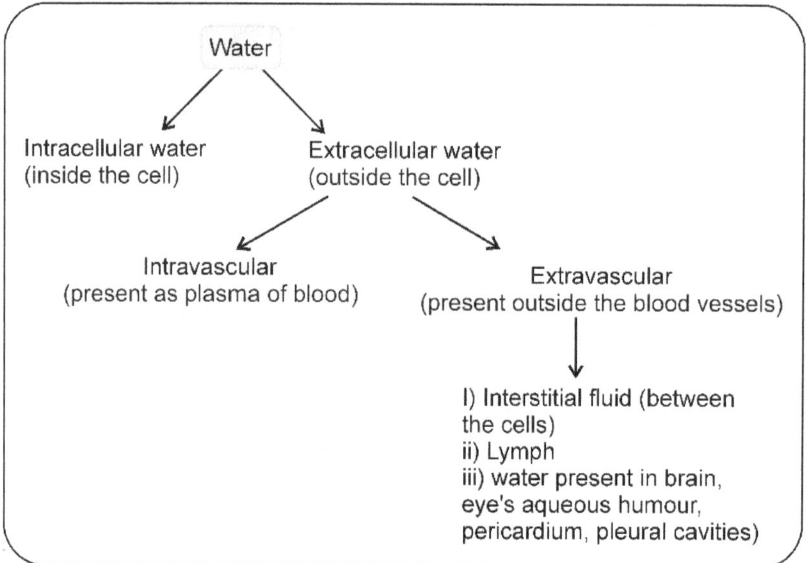

Fig. 10.1 Distribution of water in the body.

Water Turnover

Consideration is given to the external balance and internal fluxes of water turnover. Urinary water loss through the kidneys is the most prevalent method of water loss in the body. Additionally, water can be lost through diarrhoea and perspiration. Dietary intakes account for the bulk of the water consumed by the body. During metabolism, a little quantity of water is also produced. The water balance of the body can be maintained by managing fluid intake and regulating renal water excretion. External balance is the comparison of water input from and outflow to the external environment. Throughout time, input equals output, and the organism is in a condition of water balance.

Internal balance or flux refers to the transit of water across the capillaries of the body (including the generation and absorption of various transcellular fluids) and the transfer of water between interstitial and intracellular fluids. The fluid balance or body balance, or homeostasis of bodily water, is a crucial clinical component. Indicating body water homeostasis, body water turnover refers to the replenishment of body water over the course of a day or other period of time. The homeostasis of water is essential for optimum health. Body water turnover, or the gradual restoration of water lost in the body. Children under the age of 15 have a greater body water turnover than adults, while it is unknown how the ageing process impacts body water.

Among people of the same age, the rate of water turnover appears to be greater in those who exercise compared to those who are sedentary.

Electrolyte Content in Body Fluids

Electrolytes are charged particles with either a positive or negative electric charge. Electrolytes are required for healthy nervous system and muscular function, as well as a regulated internal environment. To communicate with all of the cells in the body, the brain delivers electrical impulses via nerve cells. Calcium is a necessary electrolyte for muscle contraction. Additionally, electrolytes are essential for the health of your nervous system and muscles. In addition, they keep you hydrated and help manage your pH, ensuring that the internal environment of the body is appropriate. Electrolyte imbalances may be harmful to health and even lethal in some circumstances. Electrolyte abnormalities are widespread in individuals who are highly dehydrated due to vomiting, diarrhoea, or intense sweating. Severe imbalances can wreak havoc on the body's functionality. Diet is the most effective way to acquire and maintain electrolyte balance.

There are electrolytes in the following foods:

- Fruits and vegetables are the principal dietary sources of electrolytes. In contrast, table salt is a popular source of sodium and chloride in Western diets.
- Pickled foods, cheese, and table salt are rich in sodium.
- Table salt is a source of chloride.
- Bananas, avocados, and sweet potatoes are abundant in potassium.
- Seeds and nuts provide magnesium.
- Dairy products, dairy substitutes fortified with calcium, and green leafy vegetables are all excellent sources of calcium.

Several reasons can lead to an electrolyte imbalance, including:

- Electrolyte depletion and dehydration after exercise
- Prolonged vomiting or diarrhoea; poor nutrition
- Severe dehydration acid-base imbalance (the amount of acids and alkalis in the body) chemotherapy for congestive heart failure cancer a few extra drugs, including diuretics
- Electrolytes such as bicarbonate are not required in the diet since the body spontaneously creates them.

Body Fluid Structure

The content of tissue fluid is determined by the interactions between biological tissue cells and blood. This implies that the fluid content of various physiological compartments fluctuates.

Structure of Intracellular Fluid

The majority of the cytosol, also known as the intracellular fluid, is made up of water, dissolved ions, tiny molecules, and large compounds that are water-soluble (such as proteins). The huge number of enzymes that are involved in cellular metabolism lends an extraordinary level of complexity to this mixture of minuscule molecules. These enzymes are necessary for the metabolic processes that are necessary for the survival of cells, as well as the activation and deactivation of toxic substances. The cytosol, which is mostly made up of water, accounts for around 70 percent of the total volume of a normal cell's total composition. 7.4 is the pH value found in intracellular fluid. The cytosol and the extracellular fluid are kept apart by the cell membrane throughout both the passive and active transport processes; nevertheless, the cell membrane contains channels and pumps that allow the cytosol to pass through. The quantities of other ions found in cytosol or intracellular fluid are noticeably different from those found in extracellular fluid. In addition, in comparison to the outside of the cell, the cytosol contains a far higher quantity of charged macromolecules, such as proteins and nucleic acids. In contrast to the extracellular fluid, the cytosol contains a relatively low number of sodium ions and a high concentration of potassium ions. Na^+/K ATPase pumps are the catalysts for the active movement of sodium and potassium ions, and as a consequence, they are responsible for the very accurate concentrations of these ions. These pumps transfer ions against the direction of their concentration gradients so that the ion composition of the cytosol may continue to have its fluid character.

Structure of Extracellular Fluid

Cations and anions account for the vast majority of extracellular fluid's composition. Cations contain sodium (Na^+ = 136-145 mEq/L), potassium (K^+ = 3.5-5.5 mEq/L), and calcium (Ca^{2+} = 8.4-10.5 mEq/L). Anions consist of chloride in milliequivalents per litre and hydrogen carbonate (HCO_3^- 22-26 mM). These ions are involved in the movement of water throughout the body, which they help to facilitate. Plasma is made up of dissolved proteins (albumins, fibrinogens, and globulins are the most common types of proteins), glucose, clotting factors, mineral ions (Na^+, Ca^{2+}, $Mg^{2+,}$ HCO_3^-, and other ions), hormones, and carbon dioxide (plasma being the main medium for excretory product transportation). These dissolved molecules participate in a variety of physiological activities, including as gas exchange, the activity of the immune system, and the distribution of medicines.

Structure of Transcellular Fluid

There is a large variation in the chemical make-up of the transcellular fluid that occurs according to its location. Sodium ions, chloride ions, and bicarbonate ions are all examples of the types of electrolytes that may be found in the transcellular fluid. The composition of cerebrospinal fluid is comparable to the composition of blood plasma; however, the vast majority of proteins, including albumins, are too big to pass across the blood–brain barrier. Ocular fluid, in contrast to cerebral fluid, contains a significant amount of proteins, including antibodies, despite its smaller volume. **Table 10.2** depicts dietary intake of electrolyte.

Table 10.2 Dietary intake of electrolyte

Electrolyte	Intake recommended in mg	Intake recommended in mg for people above 50 years	Intake recommended in mg for people above 70 years
Sodium	1,500	1,200	1,200
Potassium	4,700	-	-
Calcium	1,000	1,200	-
Magnesium	320 (men), 420 (women)	-	-
Chloride	2,400	2,000	1,800

Dehydration

Dehydration happens when the body lacks sufficient water to operate normally. When the body loses more water and fluids than it takes in, dehydration ensues. Low degrees of dehydration can cause headaches, fatigue, and constipation. About 75 percent of the human body is water. If it does not have access to water, it will perish. Water exists within cells, blood vessels, and between cells. A complex water management system regulates our water levels, and our thirst mechanism notifies us when we need to drink more. Although we lose water during the day through respiration, perspiration, urination, and defecation, we may replace it by consumption of fluids. If dehydration sets in, the body can also move water to areas that require it most. Dehydration may typically be treated by increasing fluid intake, but severe dehydration requires immediate medical attention.

Initial symptoms of dehydration include thirst, darker urine, and reduced urine output. In fact, the colour of urine is one of the most accurate indicators of hydration status, with clear urine suggesting adequate hydration and darker urine indicating dehydration. It is essential to keep in mind, however, that dehydration can occur without thirst, particularly in the elderly. When you are ill or the weather is hot, you should drink more water.

As a disease progresses to moderate dehydration, the following symptoms manifest:

- Dry mouth, lethargy, muscle weakness, headache, vertigo.

- Severe dehydration (loss of 10 to 15 percent of body water) is characterised by extreme versions of the foregoing symptoms, as well as dry skin, low blood pressure and increased heart rate fever delirium loss of consciousness.

Among the causes of dehydration are:

- **Vomiting and diarrhoea:** Severe, acute diarrhoea, or diarrhoea that comes suddenly and violently, can cause a rapid loss of water and electrolytes. Fluids and minerals are lost at a significantly greater rate when vomiting and diarrhoea coexist.

- **Temperature:** The higher the fever, the greater the likelihood of dehydration. If you have a fever, diarrhoea, and vomiting, the condition is much worsened.

- **Excessive perspiration:** Perspiration leads you to lose water. If you involve in rigorous exercise and do not replenish fluids as you go, you may get dehydrated. In hot, humid conditions, both the amount of sweat and the amount of fluid lost increase.

- **Increased Urination:** This might indicate undiagnosed or inadequately controlled diabetes. Certain treatments, such as diuretics and certain blood pressure medications, can also cause dehydration by increasing urination frequency.

ORT: Oral Rehydration Treatment

Oral rehydration treatment, often known as ORT, is the practise of administering a salt-and-sugar solution via the mouth in order to relieve dehydration brought on by diarrhoea. Since the World Health Organization began using ORT as its primary method of combating diarrhoea in 1978, the annual death rate among children under the age of five who suffer from acute diarrhoea has decreased from 5 million to fewer than 1 million. This has resulted in a significant reduction in the severity of the disease and the number of deaths that occur as a result of it. In underdeveloped nations, diarrhoea is the primary killer of children under the age of five and is the top cause of death overall. When a person has diarrhoea, they lose fluids in addition to electrolytes like salt and potassium from their bodies. Even if the person is still suffering from diarrhoea, ORT may still be used to refill the body in two different ways. First, sugar or glucose helps in the absorption of salt into the gut, and second, salt assists in the absorption of water into the intestinal walls. Oral rehydration therapy is not only efficient but also economic and safer.

Since then, ORT has successfully decreased diarrhea-related mortality in the developing world. Infectious diarrheas produced by viruses or entero-pathogenic bacteria, whether invasive or enterotoxigenic, take advantage of glucose-coupled sodium transport, a pathway for sodium absorption that stays largely intact in infectious diarrheas caused by viruses or enteropathogenic bacteria. Glucose enhances the transfer of salt and, to a lesser extent, water over the upper gut mucosa. Three variables impact the amount of fluid absorbed: sodium concentration, glucose concentration, and luminal fluid osmolarity. This corresponds to a sodium concentration of 40 to 90 mmol/L, a glucose concentration of 110 to 140 mmol/L (2.0 to 2.5 g/100 mL), and a sodium concentration of 40 to 90 mmol/L.

> **Chapter 11**

Introduction to Biotechnology

Biotechnology is described as "the use of organisms, cells, their components, and molecular equivalents to the production of useful products by integrating the natural and technical sciences." In 1919, Károly Ereky coined the word "biotechnology" to describe the production of goods from raw materials with the aid of living organisms. Biotechnology is a discipline of science that uses biological systems, live organisms, or their components to generate or manufacture products. The major achievement of biotechnology was the capacity to generate naturally occurring medicinal chemicals in greater quantities than could be acquired from conventional sources such as plasma, animal organs, and human cadavers. Researchers in the field of biotechnology are actively attempting to determine the underlying biological causes of disease and to intervene exactly at that level. As with the first generation of biotech medications, this may involve the production of therapeutic proteins to complement the body's natural resources or compensate for inherited deficiencies. Understanding how living creatures work at the molecular level is crucial to biotechnology, which integrates many fields like biology, physics, chemistry, mathematics, science, and technology.

In addition to producing disease-fighting products and medicines, raising food yields, and lowering greenhouse gas emissions *via* biofuels, modern biotechnology continues to make huge contributions to extending human lifespan and enhancing quality of life. In the biotechnology sector, there are several challenges to overcome. The high costs of biotech research and development are a significant factor in this. While a company commits time and money to these endeavours, there is typically limited profitability. Therefore, it is usual for biotech startups to partner with larger, more established organisations in order to achieve their research and development goals.

Development of Biotechnology

Biotechnology has existed in its most fundamental form for thousands of years, since since humans discovered how to produce bread, beer, and wine through fermentation. Biotechnology concepts were restricted to agriculture for millennia, such as increasing agricultural harvests and yields by using the finest seeds and breeding livestock.

With the discovery of microorganisms, Gregor Mendel's studies of genetics, and Pasteur and Lister's pioneering work on fermentation and microbial processes, the discipline of biotechnology began to flourish rapidly in the 19th century. The biotechnology of the early 20th century made possible Alexander Fleming's discovery of penicillin, which was thereafter produced on a wide scale in the 1940s. After World War II, a greater knowledge of cell function and molecular biology fuelled the growth of biotechnology in the 1950s. Since then, there have been significant biotechnology developments every decade. Listed here are a few of the highlights:

The three-dimensional structure of DNA was discovered in the 1950s.

In the 1960s, insulin was synthesised and measles, mumps, and rubella vaccines were created.

In the 1970s, significant advancements were achieved in DNA research.

In the 1980s, the first drugs and vaccines produced from biotechnology were created to treat diseases such as cancer and hepatitis B.

In the 1990s, more genes were found, and for the first time in decades, new treatments for multiple sclerosis and cystic fibrosis were introduced.

The completion of the human genome sequence in the 1990s, allowing scientists throughout the world to research novel therapies for hereditary disorders such as cancer, heart disease, and Alzheimer's disease.

Current Status of Biotechnology

The biotechnology industry has grown exponentially since the 1990s. Gilead Sciences, Amgen, Biogen Idec, and Celgene are just a handful of the medical industry's titans that have arisen. On the opposite end of the spectrum are thousands of small, vibrant biotech enterprises, many of which are engaged in various medical sector components, such as drug development, genomics, or proteomics, while others are involved in bioremediation, biofuels, and food products.

Pharmaceutical Firms vs Biotechnology Firms

Both biotechnology and pharmaceutical industries produce medicines. In contrast, biotechnology companies' pharmaceuticals are derived from living creatures, whereas pharmaceutical companies' therapies are often chemically based.

Companies that do research and development employing both biotechnology and chemicals are referred to as biopharma. Examples of biopharmaceutical products include plastic, laundry detergent, immunizations, beer, and wine. The most prevalent products sold by pharmaceutical industries are drugs and supplements.

Biotechnology s utilise the activities of living organisms to create innovative problem-solving solutions. Utilizing DNA has led to the development of pest-resistant crops, biofuels such as ethanol, and gene cloning.

The Cleveland Clinic has identified the top 10 pharmaceutical medical discoveries for 2021. Among these were calcitonin gene-related peptide (CGRP) inhibitors for the treatment of prostate cancer and a new family of migraine drugs called calcitonin gene-related peptide inhibitors (CGRP). In addition, vacuum-induced uterine tamponade, a novel therapy for postpartum bleeding, will be of great help to women in developing nations with limited access to other treatments.

Exelixis, Novavax, and Regeneron Pharmaceuticals are prominent biotechnology companies.

Applications of Biotechnology

Bioinformatics, sometimes referred to as "gold biotechnology," is an interdisciplinary discipline that use computing methods to tackle biological issues and enables the rapid organisation and analysis of biological data. Functional genomics, structural genomics, and proteomics, as well as the biotechnology and pharmaceutical sectors, rely heavily on bioinformatics.

Blue biotechnology refers to the exploitation of marine resources to develop goods and industrial applications.

This area of biotechnology is particularly prevalent in the refining and combustion industries, with a concentration on the production of bio-oils from microphotosynthetic algae.

The application of biotechnology to agricultural operations constitutes green biotechnology. Micropropagation can be used, for instance, to select and domesticate plants. The production of transgenic plants that can flourish in specified situations with (or without) pesticides is another illustration.

Red biotechnology refers to the use of biotechnology in the medical and pharmaceutical industries, as well as for health preservation. The creation of vaccines and antibiotics, as well as regenerative treatments, the production of artificial organs, and novel disease diagnostics.

Industrial biotechnology, sometimes known as white biotechnology, is the application of biotechnology to industrial processes.

"Yellow biotechnology" refers to the use of biotechnology in the food industry, including the fermentation of wine, cheese, and beer (brewing).

Gray biotechnology term is devoted to environmental applications, with an emphasis on the preservation of biodiversity and the elimination of pollution.

Brown biotechnology is connected to the management of arid environments and deserts.

Violet biotechnology is concerned with biotechnology's legal, ethical, and philosophical challenges. One application is the development of seeds that can withstand the harsh environmental conditions of dry locations. This application is related to innovation, agriculture technology development, and resource management.

Dark biotechnology is related with bioterrorism, biological weapons, and biowarfare, in which germs and chemicals are utilised to infect humans, livestock, and crops in order to cause sickness and death.

Biotechnology has several medical applications, including drug development and manufacture, pharmacogenomics, and genetic testing (or genetic screening).

By correlating gene expression or single-nucleotide polymorphisms with a drug's efficacy or toxicity, researchers in this field investigate the impact of genetic variation on patients' pharmacological responses. The objective of pharmacogenomics is to develop strategies for optimising pharmaceutical therapy based on a patient's genotype in order to achieve maximum efficacy with minimal adverse effects.

> **Chapter 12**

Organ Function Tests

These are the tests carried out to assess whether a particular organ is functioning normally or not.

1. Kidneys

The kidneys are one of the most essential organs in the body. Kidney failure can cause serious illness or even death. Each kidney's structure and function are exceedingly complex. Creatinine and urea are two important waste products that can be detected in the blood. The "results" of blood tests represent the function of the kidney. When both kidneys fail, blood levels of creatinine and urea are elevated. The second most important function of the kidney is fluid balance regulation, which entails excreting excess water as urine while retaining the minimum quantity of water required for survival.

Consequently, the kidneys perform two essential functions: flushing out harmful and deadly waste products and regulating the balance of water, fluids, minerals, and chemicals, such as electrolytes such as sodium and potassium. Approximately one million filtration units known as nephrons comprise each kidney. Each nephron consists of a filter known as the glomerulus and a tubule. The glomerulus filters the blood, whereas the tubule restores necessary elements to the blood while eliminating wastes. Urine production begins with the filtration of 125 mL of urine per minute by the glomeruli. In only 24 hours, 180 litres of pee may be generated. In addition to waste products, electrolytes, and harmful molecules, it includes glucose and other helpful chemicals.

As blood reaches each nephron, it enters a collection of small blood vessels known as the glomerulus. Through the glomerulus's thin walls, smaller molecules, wastes, and fluids, primarily water, can enter the tubule. For example, proteins and blood cells are bigger molecules that remain in the blood vessel. The tubule removes wastes and returns necessary chemicals to the circulation. In close proximity to the tubule lies an artery. As the filtered fluid travels down the tubule, the blood vessel reabsorbs virtually all of the water, as well as the minerals and nutrients required by the organism. Tubules contribute to the elimination of excess acid from the circulation. Therefore, urine is produced from the fluid and wastes remaining in the tubule. Before being ejected, urine generated by the kidneys passes via the ureters, urinary bladder, and urethra.

The kidneys are chemical factories that perform the following functions: removing waste from the body, removing drugs from the body, and regulating the body's fluid balance.

Red blood cell production is regulated; blood pressure-regulating hormones are released; an active form of vitamin D is produced; and red blood cell production is regulated.

Major Kidney Functions

Protein is present in the food we consume. The body needs protein for development and repair. However, when the body utilises protein, waste products are created. The collection and retention of these waste products resembles the retention of poison by the body. Each kidney filters blood and toxic wastes before excreting them via urine. In the event of renal failure, the kidneys are unable to eliminate extra water. The reason of swelling is an excess of water in the body. In addition to maintaining proper body fluid composition, the kidneys regulate minerals and substances such as sodium, potassium, hydrogen, calcium, phosphorus, magnesium, and bicarbonate.

- Changes in sodium levels can alter a person's mental state, whereas changes in potassium levels can have significant effects on the heart's rhythm and muscular function.

- Normal calcium and phosphorus levels are necessary for healthy bones and teeth. In addition, many hormones (renin, angiotensin, aldosterone, prostaglandin, and others) are generated by the kidneys to help balance water and salt in the body, which is essential for maintaining proper blood pressure control.

- In patients with renal illness, changes in hormone synthesis and salt and water management can lead to hypertension.

The kidneys also create erythropoietin, which contributes in the production of red blood cells (RBC). Kidney failure decreases erythropoietin production, which in turn reduces RBC production, resulting in low haemoglobin levels (anemia). Due to this, the haemoglobin count of people with renal failure does not improve despite therapy with iron and vitamin supplements. Vitamin D is converted by the kidneys into its active form, which is necessary for calcium absorption from the food, bone and tooth development, and bone health. When you have renal failure, your levels of active vitamin D decrease, causing your bones to stop developing and become brittle. Kidney failure can impede the growth of children.

Evaluation of the Kidney's Functioning

Kidneys in good health eliminate wastes and extra fluid from the bloodstream. Blood and urine tests can be performed to evaluate the health of the kidneys and the rate at which waste is removed. Additionally, urine tests can detect abnormal protein leakage from the kidneys, a sign of renal disease. Here is a summary of the several tests used to evaluate kidney function.

- **Testing of Blood:** Creatinine is a by product of muscle wear and tear. The concentration of creatinine in the blood changes with age and body size. A creatinine level of greater than 1.2 in females and greater than 1.4 in males may suggest improper renal function. As renal disease progresses, creatinine levels in the blood grow.

Glomerular Filtration Rate (GFR): This test measures the kidneys' ability to eliminate waste and excess fluid from the circulation. Multiplying the blood creatinine level by the patient's age and gender yields the creatinine clearance. Normal GFR fluctuates with ageing (as you get older it can decrease). GFR must be greater than 90 to be deemed normal. The kidneys are not working adequately if the GFR is less than 60. Once the GFR goes below 15, the likelihood of requiring dialysis or a kidney transplant to treat renal failure increases significantly.

Blood Urea Nitrogen (BUN): The digestion of protein in the food you eat leads to the production of urea nitrogen in your body. The levels of BUN should fall around between 7 and 20. BUN levels tend to rise in conjunction with a decline in renal function.

- **Urine Examination:** A urine test that lasts for 24 hours can provide a more accurate picture of how well your kidneys are functioning and how much protein is lost into your urine. This test measures how much urine your kidneys produce in a day. Additionally, it can determine how much urine your kidneys produce in a day.

The urinalysis test known as the dipstick test involves dipping a strip that has been chemically treated into a urine sample. When abnormalities such as excess protein, blood, pus, germs, or sugar are present, the strip will change colour. These abnormalities will trigger the change. An accurate diagnosis of chronic kidney disease, diabetes, bladder infection, and kidney stones may be made by urinalysis.

Protein in Urine: Dipstick testing may be used either as part of a comprehensive urinalysis or on its own to determine the presence of protein in the urine. A condition known as proteinuria is characterised by an abnormally high concentration of protein in the urine. A positive result from a standard dipstick test (1+ or higher) has to be validated by either a more specialised dipstick test, such as an albumin-specific dipstick, or a quantitative measurement, such as the ratio of albumin to creatinine.

This is a more sensitive dipstick test for microalbuminuria, which means that it has the potential to detect a very little amount of albumin, which is a protein that may be found in urine. People who are at an elevated risk of developing renal disease, such as those who have diabetes or high blood pressure, should undertake this test or an albumin-to-creatinine ratio test if a normal dipstick test for proteinuria is negative. Both of these tests may be found online.

Ratio of Albumin to Creatinine (ACR): The kidneys' function may be determined from the results of this urine test. The amount of albumin found in the urine is the first thing that is measured. Albumin is the kind of protein that is seen in urine the most often. The presence of albumin in the urine may be an indication that the kidneys are not working as they should be. The ACR may be determined by dividing the amount of urine albumin by the amount of urine creatinine in order to complete the calculation. Values of the ACR that are lower than 30 are regarded to be normal. Significantly high albuminuria is indicated by an ACR between 30 and 300. When the ACR is more than 300, significant albuminuria is present.

Elimination of Creatinine: The muscles of the body generate creatinine as a by product of normal wear and strain. The creatinine clearance test compares the creatinine level in your blood to the creatinine level in a 24-hour urine sample in order to establish how much trash your kidneys filter out per minute.

2. Liver

The liver is the biggest solid organ in the body. It removes toxins from the bloodstream, controls blood clotting, and carries out hundreds of other essential functions. The liver is located above the stomach, the right kidney, and the intestines in the upper right quadrant of the abdominal cavity, just below the diaphragm. The liver is a dark reddish-brown organ that weighs around 3 pounds and has a conical shape. The liver receives blood from two distinct sources, which include:

The hepatic artery carries oxygenated blood into the liver.

The hepatic portal vein carries nutrient-rich blood into the liver.

At any one time, the liver is responsible for storing around one pint, or thirteen percent, of the body's total blood supply. The liver is divided into two sections called lobes. Each one is made up of eight segments and has a thousand lobules (small lobes). These lobules are linked to one another by means of smaller ducts (tubes) in order to form the common hepatic duct, which in turn connects to channels of a greater diameter. The bile that is produced by liver cells is sent to both the gallbladder and the duodenum through the common hepatic duct (the first portion of the small intestine). The liver is a vital organ that conducts over 500 human functions. The liver removes waste items and foreign chemicals from the bloodstream, regulates blood sugar levels, and produces essential nutrients. Here are some of its most important characteristics:

- Filters Blood: The liver removes toxins, byproducts, and other harmful compounds from all blood leaving the stomach and intestines.

- Regulates Amino Acids: Protein synthesis requires amino acids. The liver regulates the concentration of amino acids in the circulation.

- Vitamin K, which can only be absorbed with the aid of bile, a fluid generated by the liver, is utilised to manufacture blood clotting coagulants.

- Protects Against Infections: As part of this process, the liver filters the bloodstream and removes microorganisms.

- Large quantities of vitamins A, D, E, K, and B_{12}, as well as iron and copper, are stored in the liver.

The liver accumulates and stores excess glucose (sugar) in the circulation. As required, it can convert glycogen to glucose.

- Produces bile, which assists in waste removal and fat digestion in the small intestine during digestion.

- Produces blood plasma proteins.

- Produces cholesterol and unique proteins that facilitate the transport of lipids throughout the body.

- Haemoglobin is processed so that the iron it contains may be used (the liver stores iron).

- Ammonia is transformed to the less poisonous urea (urea is one of the end products of protein metabolism that is excreted in the urine).

- Removes from the circulation medicines and other potentially dangerous substances.

- Prevents blood clotting

- Produces immune factors and eliminates pathogens from circulation to combat disease.

- A damaged or failing liver that clears bilirubin (excess bilirubin causes yellowing of the skin and eyes) can have dangerous or even deadly consequences.

The following instances illustrate liver disease:

- Fascioliasis is a parasitic infection caused by a liver fluke, a parasitic worm that can remain latent in the liver for months or even years. Fascioliasis is a tropical illness. Toxins, alcohol, and hepatitis are a few potential causes of this condition. As the functioning of liver cells deteriorates, fibrosis may finally result in liver failure.

- Hepatitis refers to an infection of the liver that may be caused by viruses, toxins, or an autoimmune reaction. A liver that is inflamed is one of the signs. In many instances, the liver is capable of self-repair, but in extreme situations, liver failure can occur.

Consuming high quantities of alcohol over an extended period of time is the cause of alcoholic liver damage. This is the most prevalent cause of cirrhosis across the globe.

- PSC (primary sclerosing cholangitis) is a destructive inflammatory disease of the bile ducts that destroys them. It is incurable and its cause is unclear, however it is presumed to be an autoimmune disorder.

- Fatty liver disease is most frequently linked to obesity or alcohol intake. In fatty liver disease, fat vacuoles form in liver cells. The condition is called non-alcoholic fatty liver disease if it is not caused by excessive alcohol consumption (NAFLD).

- Genetics, medications, and a high-fructose diet are the most prevalent reasons. It is the most prevalent liver ailment in wealthy nations and has been related to insulin resistance. If NAFLD progresses, the condition nonalcoholic steatohepatitis (NASH) may develop. NASH is known to develop cirrhosis of the liver.

- Gilbert's syndrome is an inherited illness that affects 3 to 12 percent of the population. Bilirubin has not been entirely broken down. Mild jaundice is a perfectly innocuous disease that can develop.

The two most common types of liver cancer are hepatocellular carcinoma and cholangiocarcinoma. Hepatitis and alcohol use are the main culprits. It is the sixth most prevalent form of cancer and the second largest cause of cancer-related death.

Tests to Assess the Functions of Liver and their Clinical Significances

Serum bilirubin test: This test determines the amounts of bilirubin that are present in the blood. The bilirubin that is produced by the liver is then eliminated by the body via the bile. An elevated level of bilirubin may be an indicator of a problem with the liver's ability to digest bile or with the flow of bile itself.

Serum albumin: This test may assist in the diagnosis of liver illness by determining the quantity of albumin (a protein found in the blood) that is present inside the body. Low albumin levels might be an indication that something is wrong with the liver's function.

The prothrombin time (PT) test is formally known as the international normalised ratio (INR): This test determines how long blood takes to clot. Vitamin K and a protein produced by the liver are required for blood clotting. Prolonged clotting could be a sign of liver illness or a lack of particular clotting factors.

Alkaline phosphatase test in the blood: The level of alkaline phosphatase (an enzyme) in the blood is measured using this test. Alkaline phosphatase is found in a variety of tissues, with the liver, biliary tract, and bone having the largest quantities. This test can be used to determine how well the liver is working and to look for liver abnormalities that could cause biliary blockage, such as tumours or abscesses.

Alanine transaminase test (ALT): The level of alanine aminotransferase is measured in this test. This is a liver enzyme that is released into the bloodstream when acute liver cell injury occurs. This test can be used to examine liver function and/or to determine the effectiveness of treatment for acute liver disease such hepatitis.

Aspartate transaminase test (AST): Aspartate transaminase is measured in this test. After liver or heart problems, an enzyme present in the liver, kidneys, pancreas, heart, skeletal muscle, and red blood cells is released into the bloodstream. After acute liver cell injury, this enzyme is released into the bloodstream.

Gamma-glutamyl transpeptidase test: The gamma-glutamyl transpeptidase level is measured in this test. The liver, pancreas, and biliary tract all produce this enzyme. This test is commonly used to evaluate liver function, provide information about liver disorders, and detect alcohol consumption.

Test for lactic dehydrogenase: This test can detect tissue damage and may help with liver disease diagnosis. Lactic dehydrogenase is a protein that breaks down lactose (also called an isoenzyme). It is engaged in the metabolic process of the organism. This is, however, a very broad liver test. It is rarely used to diagnose liver disease.

Test for 5'-nucleotidase: The levels of 5'- nucleotidase are measured in this test (an enzyme specific to the liver). The level of 5'- nucleotidase is higher in people who have liver problems, especially those who have cholestasis. The creation of bile is disrupted, and the flow of bile is obstructed.

3. Lipid Profile Tests

The number of lipids (fat molecules) that are present in a person's circulation may be measured using a blood test known as a lipid profile test. It is possible for cholesterol and triglycerides to accumulate in the blood vessels and arteries when there is an excessive amount of cholesterol and triglycerides in the circulation. This may lead to tissue damage and an increased risk of cardiovascular disease. As a consequence of this, lipid profile tests are administered to both children and adults in order to determine their respective risks of developing cardiovascular diseases such as heart disease, heart attack (myocardial infarction), and stroke.

A lipid panel analyses a blood sample for five different types of lipids, including:

- Overall cholesterol level may be represented by total cholesterol, which is a mix of LDL-C, VLDL-C, and HDL-C levels.

- LDL cholesterol, sometimes known as "bad cholesterol," is a kind of cholesterol that has a high concentration of low-density lipoprotein (LDL). It is possible for it to accumulate in the blood arteries, which raises the risk of heart disease. Fewer than 100 milligrammes per deciliter (mg/dL) for low-density lipoprotein (LDL) cholesterol; less than 70 milligrammes per deciliter (mg/dL) for diabetics.

- VLDL cholesterol, also known as very low-density lipoprotein cholesterol, is a kind of cholesterol that is generally seen in very tiny levels in blood samples taken when the subject is fasting. This is because VLDL cholesterol is mostly formed from food that has been recently consumed. If there is an increase in this kind of cholesterol in a sample taken when the individual is fasting, this may signal that there is an issue with lipid metabolism.

- HDL cholesterol, also known as high-density lipoprotein cholesterol, is referred to as the "good cholesterol." HDL cholesterol is the kind of cholesterol that is found in the body. It helps to reduce the amount of bad LDL cholesterol that builds up in the blood vessels.

- Triglycerides are a kind of fat that may be obtained by one's diet. Triglyceride levels that are too high in the blood have been related to cardiovascular disease as well as inflammation in the pancreas. Triglycerides should be less than 150 mg/dL.

- For each of the four standard tests in a lipid panel, the ideal level (measured in milligrams per decilitre of blood — mg/dL) is as follows:

4. The results may be classed as borderline-, intermediate-, or high-risk for cardiovascular disorders if they are greater or lower than the target range. Higher-than-normal total cholesterol, LDL, and triglyceride levels, as well as lower-than-normal HDL levels, can all raise risk of cardiovascular disease. **Table 12.1** depicts the range of cholesterol present in the body and their effects.

Table 12.1 The range of cholesterol present in the body and their effects.

Total cholesterol	Condition
< 200 mg/dL	Optimum
Within range 210-239 mg/dL	Slightly towards high range
> 240 mg/dL	High

LDL cholesterol values (in mg/dL)	Condition
<70	Best for people who have coronary artery disease — including a history of heart attacks, angina, stents or coronary bypass.
<100	Optimal for individuals with a history of diabetes or coronary heart disease risk. For persons with simple coronary artery disease, this is close to ideal.
Within range 100-129	If there is no coronary artery disease, almost optimum. High if coronary artery disease is present.
Within range 130-159	Borderline high if coronary artery disease is not diagnosed. High if coronary artery disease is diagnosed.
Within range 160-189	If there is no coronary artery disease, it is high. Extremely high if coronary artery disease is present.
>190	Very high

HDL cholesterol (mg/dL)	Condition
<40	poor
40-59, men 50-59, women	better
>60	best

Triglycerides (mg/dL)	Condition
<150	Optimal
Within range 150-199	Slightly high
Within range 200-499	High
>500	Higher

> **Chapter 13**

Introduction to Pathology Blood and Urine

The examination of organs, tissues, and physiological fluids is done in pathology, which is the study of disease as well as its diagnosis (autopsies). It is possible to trace the origins of pathology all the way back to the earliest applications of the scientific method to the field of medicine, which took place during the Islamic Golden Age and the Italian Renaissance, respectively, in the Middle East and Western Europe. These two historical periods are considered to be the beginnings of Western civilization. In the early third century B.C., the ancient Greek physicians Herophilus of Chalcedon and Erasistratus of Chios performed the first systematic human dissections. Arabian physician Avenzoar (1091–1161) was the first documented physician to perform postmortem dissections. The production of lesions is referred to as **pathogenesis of disease**. The patient's perceptions of the lesion's functional consequences are symptoms, whereas the clinician's observations are physical signs. The **diagnosis** is the clinical value of the morphological and functional alterations as well as the findings of additional examinations that serve to determine the precise nature of the problem. It is generally accepted that Rudolf Virchow (1821–1902) is the father of microscopic pathology. The various branches of pathology includes:

- **Anatomical pathology** is the study of anatomical features, such as tissue taken from the body, or even the full body in the case of an autopsy, with the purpose of diagnosing illness and increasing our knowledge of it. The study of anatomical pathology could include looking at cells under a microscope, but it also encompasses a more in-depth investigation of organs (e.g a ruptured spleen). In addition to this, analysis of the chemical properties and immunological markers of cells is included. Several main subgroups of anatomical pathology exist:

- **Surgical pathology** is the study of surgically removed tissues. Examining a little portion of tumour tissue to identify whether the tumour is malignant (cancerous) or benign and make a diagnosis is a frequent example. This process is known as a biopsy.

- **Histopathology** is the microscopic study of cells that have been dyed to make them visible or easier to observe. Frequently, antibodies are employed to identify distinct cellular components with distinct hues of dye or fluorescence. After the microscope's broad adoption in pathology, several techniques for preserving and colouring tissue were devised.

- **Cytopathology** is the study of tiny groups of cells acquired from biological fluids or scrapings, such as those retrieved after a Pap smear. A Pap smear can identify cervical cancer and some infections. The cervix is swabbed to collect cells, which are subsequently processed and viewed under a microscope for abnormalities.

- **Clinical pathology** identifies illness by analysing physiological fluids and tissues in the laboratory. For instance, the chemical components of blood may be studied, as well as the cells and any microbes, such as bacteria, present in a sample. Clinical pathology is sometimes referred to as laboratory medicine on occasion. Important varieties include the following:

- **Clinical chemistry** or **chemical pathology** involves the chemical examination of body fluids by testing and microscopy. Chemical pathology often involves the study of blood and its immunological components, such as white blood cells.

- **Hematology,** like chemical pathology, is concerned with the study of blood, but it focuses more on detecting particular blood illnesses. Additionally, haematologists examine the lymph system and bone marrow, which are also components of the hematopoietic system.

- **Immunology** or **immunopathology** is the study of abnormalities of the immune system. It covers immunological reactions to foreign molecules, allergies, immunodeficiencies, and organ transplant rejection.

- **Molecular pathology** is the study of tissue and cell disorders at the molecular level. It is a wide category that refers to the investigation of illness in any organ or tissue of the body by analysing the chemicals present in cells. It may incorporate both anatomical and clinical pathology. In molecular pathology, methods such as polymerase chain reaction (PCR) to amplify DNA, fluorescence labelling, karyotype imaging of chromosomes, and DNA microarrays are utilised (small samples of DNA placed onto biochips).

Thus, pathology is concerned with disease processes, including aetiology, pathogenesis, and clinical manifestations in animals, and attempts to explain what went wrong. It links the fundamental information acquired in anatomy, histology, physiology, and biochemistry with clinical issues to aid in illness diagnosis, treatment, prevention, and control.

Lymphocytes

White blood cells comprise lymphocytes. They are an essential component of our immune system. Approximately 20% to 40% of your white blood cells are lymphocytes. 600 to 700 red blood cells are accompanied by one white blood cell. The white blood cells operate like body's army. White blood cells are spread throughout our body, but when a pathogen or virus invades, they instantly assemble to repel it. Lymphocytes are derived from bone marrow stem cells. Some of these cells then go to the thymus, where they develop into T cells. Others stay in the bone marrow and transform into B cells. After encountering an antigen, some lymphocytes transform into memory cells. When these memory cells encounter an antigen for the second time, they react swiftly and specifically. Vaccines can prevent some diseases for this reason. Normal lymphocyte levels vary with ageing. The typical lymphocyte count for people is between 1,000 to 4,800 per microliter of blood. Between 3,500 to 9,500 lymphocytes per microliter of blood are seen in children.

Two kinds of lymphocytes are as follows:

- **B cells (B lymphocytes).** They produce antibodies. Antibodies can eliminate foreign chemicals or mark them for destruction.

- **T cells (T lymphocytes).** These lymphocytes eliminate any infected or malignant cells in the body.

B cells are responsible for producing antibodies, which are proteins generated by the immune system to combat antigens, which are foreign substances. Each B cell produces a unique antibody. Each antibody is designed to destroy a certain antigen. The matching procedure is analogous to how a key fits into a lock. T cells aid the body in destroying cancer cells and regulate the immune response to foreign chemicals. They do this by eliminating cells in the body that have been infected by viruses or transformed into malignant cells.

A third type of lymphocyte, known as an NK cell or natural killer cell, originates from the same location as B and T cells. NK cells are specialised in eliminating cancer cells and virus-infected cells and respond rapidly to a variety of foreign chemicals.

There are several varieties of B cells and T cells, each with a distinct function inside the body and immune system.

Memory B cells circulate throughout the body in order to initiate a rapid antibody response when they detect a foreign material. They persist in the body for decades and transform into memory cells that recall antigens and enable the immune system to respond more quickly to subsequent attacks **(Fig. 13.1)**.

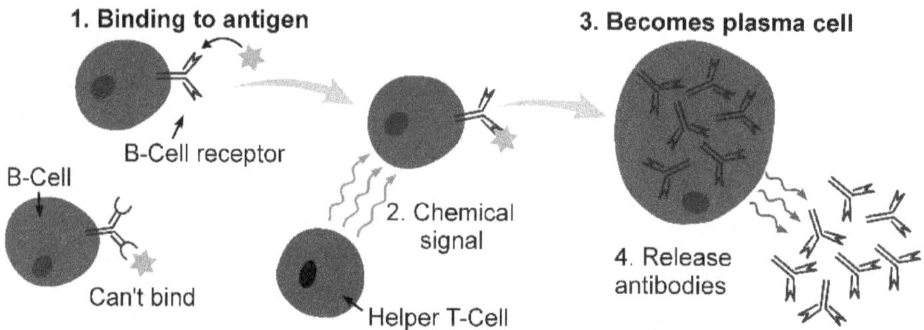

Fig. 13.1 Role of B cells and T cells.

Restrictive B cells: Bregs, or regulatory B cells, account for a modest percentage of B cells in healthy individuals. Although small in number, they play an essential function. Bregs provide beneficial anti-inflammatory actions on the body and inhibit inflammatory lymphocytes. In addition, they interact with a variety of other immune cells and stimulate the creation of regulatory T cells, or Tregs.

Plasma cells: Plasma cells are B cells that have undergone terminal differentiation and are responsible for antibody-mediated immunity. Terminally differentiated cells are cells that have grown so specialised that they are no longer able to divide.

T cells: Several kinds of T cells exist:

Killer T cells: Killer, or cytotoxic, T cells examine the surface of bodily cells to determine if they have gotten infected with pathogens or transformed into malignant cells. If so, these cells are eliminated.

Helper T cells: Helper T cells "assist" other immune system cells in initiating and regulating the immune response to foreign chemicals. There are several kinds of helper T cells, some of which are more efficient than others against certain types of pathogens.

Regulatory T cells, often known as Tregs: Tregs regulate or inhibit other immune system cells. They have both positive and negative consequences. They maintain tolerance to pathogens, inhibit autoimmunity, and control inflammation. However, they can also inhibit the immune system's ability to combat specific antigens and malignancies.

Natural killer T cells: Natural killer T cells are a heterogeneous population of T cells that share traits with natural killer cells. They can impact other immune cells and regulate immunological responses against things that induce an immune response within the body.

Counts of T cells that exceed the usual range may suggest any of the following conditions:

- STIs, such as syphilis, are sexually transmitted diseases.
- Infection with a virus, such as infectious mononucleosis.
- Infectious parasitic diseases, such as toxoplasmosis.
- White blood cell malignancy, acute lymphoblastic leukaemia of T-cells.
- multiple myeloma (cancer of the blood, starting in the bone marrow).

B cell counts above the norm may indicate:

- Leukemia lymphocytic chronique (CLL).
- Multiple myeloma.
- A kind of cancer known as Waldenstrom macroglobulinemia or Waldenstrom's disease.
- A disease with acquired T cell depletion, such as HIV.
- A variety of cancer.
- DiGeorge syndrome.

B cell levels below the norm may indicate:

- B-cell acute lymphoblastic leukaemia
- HIV or another immune-compromising condition
- DiGeorge syndrome.

Blood levels of lymphocytes that are elevated often suggest an infection or other inflammatory disorder. An increase in lymphocytes indicates that these white blood cells are mobilising to clear the body of a pathogen that might cause illness. Sometimes dangerous conditions, such as blood or lymphatic system malignancies, can generate high lymphocyte numbers.

Platelets

Platelets are tiny blood cells that aid in the formation of blood clots to stop bleeding **(Fig. 13.2)**. When a blood artery is compromised, it sends messages to the platelets. The platelets then rush to the damaged area and form a plug (clot) to repair it. Platelets, also known as thrombocytes, are a blood component whose purpose (together with the coagulation factors) is to initiate a blood clot in response to blood vessel injury-induced bleeding. Platelets are cytoplasmic fragments generated from megakaryocytes of the bone marrow or lung that enter the bloodstream. Inactivated platelets in circulation are biconvex discoid (lens-shaped) formations with a maximum diameter of 2–3 µm. Adhesion refers to the process of spreading over the surface of a damaged blood artery in order to halt bleeding. This is due to the fact that when platelets get to the location of the damage, they generate tentacles that assist them cling to one another. In addition, they emit chemical signals to recruit other platelets. Additional platelets adhere to the clot through a process known as aggregation. Platelets are produced with white and red blood cells in the bone marrow. Typically, medical professionals refer to a clot as a thrombus. Once platelets are produced and circulated in the circulation, they have a lifespan of eight to ten days.

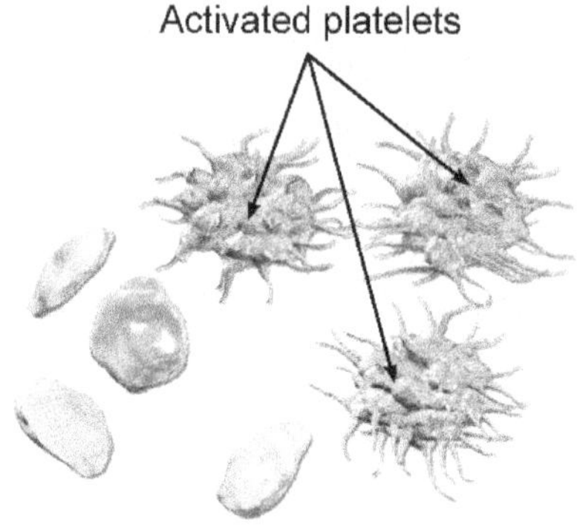

Fig. 13.2 Diagram of platelets.

Disorders

- **Thrombocytopenia** refers to disorder when the bone marrow produces an insufficiency of platelets or platelets will be eliminated. If platelet count is found to be too low, bleeding under the skin might manifest as a bruise or it might occur inside as internal bleeding or it might occur externally through a wound that will not stop bleeding or a nosebleed. If the individuals have platelet counts more than 1 million, it may result in bleeding, formation of blood clots that obstruct blood flow to the brain or heart. Several medications, cancer, liver disease, pregnancy, infections, and an aberrant immune system are some of the examples.

- **Thrombocytopenia secondary** is another disorder induced by an excess of platelets. More prevalent than primary thrombocytosis is secondary thrombocytosis. It is not caused by an issue with the bone marrow. In contrast, another disease or condition promotes the bone marrow to produce more platelets. Infection, inflammation, some forms of malignancy, and adverse drug responses are among the causes. Generally, symptoms associated with thrombocytopenia secondary not significant. The platelet count returns to normal when the underlying disease improves.

- **Poor platelet function:** A number of uncommon disorders are associated with impaired platelet function. This indicates that the platelet count is normal, but their function is impaired. Aspirin and other medications can cause this. It is essential to understand which medications impact platelets.

Platelets are little but vital blood cells that assist the body manage bleeding. A simple blood test is sufficient to determine whether or not your platelet count is normal.

Erythrocyte: By far the most prevalent produced constituent is the erythrocyte, also known as a red blood cell (or RBC) (**Fig. 13.3**). There are millions of erythrocytes and just thousands of leukocytes in a single drop of blood. Men have roughly 5.4 million erythrocytes per microliter (µL) of blood, whereas women have approximately 4.8 million per µL. It is believed that erythrocytes constitute around 25 percent of all body cells. The basic roles of erythrocytes are to carry oxygen from the lungs to the tissues of the body and to transfer carbon dioxide waste from the tissues to the lungs for expiration. Erythrocytes continue to exist inside the vascular system. Although leukocytes normally leave the blood vessels to carry out their protective duties, erythrocyte migration from the blood channels is aberrant. Erythrocytes are biconcave discs whose centres are quite shallow. This configuration maximises the ratio of surface area to volume, hence improving gas exchange. It also allows them to fold up while passing through tiny blood channels.

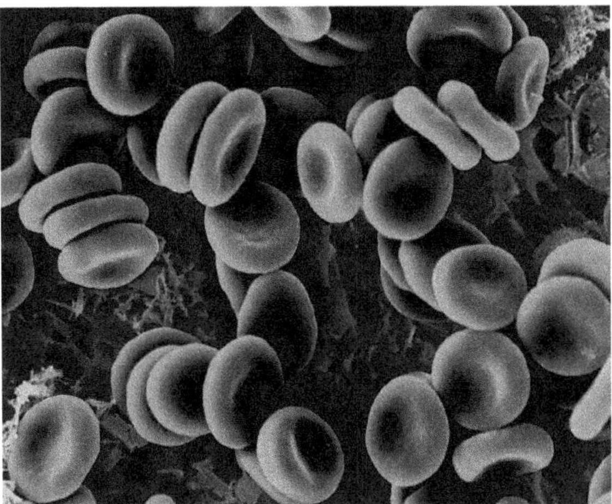

Fig. 13.3 Diagram of red blood cells.

The bone marrow produces erythrocytes at a stunning pace of more than 2 million cells per second. A number of necessary quantities of raw materials must be present for this production to occur. These include glucose, lipids, and amino acids, all of which are vital to the formation and maintenance of all cells. However, the formation of erythrocytes also requires certain trace elements:

- **Iron:** Each heme group in a haemoglobin molecule includes an ion of the trace mineral iron, as previously stated. Less than twenty percent of the iron we ingest is absorbed on average. Heme iron, which is found in animal foods like meat, poultry, and fish, is absorbed more efficiently than non-heme iron, which is found in plant foods. Iron becomes a component of the body's total iron pool upon absorption. Iron is stored in the bone marrow, liver, and spleen as the protein complexes ferritin and hemosiderin. Ferroportin carries iron through the plasma membranes of intestinal cells and from its storage sites into tissue fluid, where it is absorbed into the blood. Iron is freed from storage, attached to transferrin, and transported to the red marrow, where it connects to erythrocyte precursors when EPO drives erythrocyte formation. Globin, the protein component of haemoglobin, is degraded into amino acids, which are then sent to the bone marrow for use in the synthesis of new erythrocytes. Hemoglobin that is not phagocytosed is degraded in the circulation, releasing alpha and beta chains that are filtered by the kidneys. The iron present in the heme part of haemoglobin can be retained in the liver or spleen, typically as ferritin or hemosiderin, or transported to the red bone marrow via transferrin for recycling into new erythrocytes. The non-iron part of heme gets degraded into the green pigment biliverdin and ultimately the yellow pigment bilirubin. Bilirubin attaches to albumin and travels in the blood to the liver, which utilises it to produce bile, a substance that aids in the emulsification of dietary lipids. Bacteria in the large intestine separate bilirubin from bile and convert it into urobilinogen and eventually stercobilin. It is afterwards removed in the faeces. These bacteria are normally eliminated by broad-spectrum antibiotics, which may also affect the colour of faeces. Additionally, the kidneys release into the urine any circulating bilirubin and other metabolic by-products such as urobilin. In various circumstances, breakdown pigments resulting from the degradation of haemoglobin can be seen. At the location of an injury, biliverdin produced by damaged RBCs is responsible for part of the vivid colours associated with bruising. With a failing liver, bilirubin cannot be properly eliminated from circulation, resulting in the jaundice-associated yellowing of the skin. Stercobilins in faeces are responsible for the characteristic brown hue of this excrement. And the yellow colour of urine is due to urobilin.

- **Copper:** Copper, a trace mineral, is present in two plasma proteins, hephaestin and ceruloplasmin. Without them, haemoglobin production would be ineffective. Hephaestin, which is found in intestinal villi, promotes iron absorption by intestinal cells. Copper is transported through ceruloplasmin. Both allow for the oxidation of iron from $Fe2+$ to $Fe3+$, a form that may be coupled to its transport protein, transferrin, for delivery to body cells. In a situation of copper shortage, the transit of iron for heme production is diminished, and iron can accumulate in tissues, leading to organ damage.

- **Zinc:** As a coenzyme, the trace mineral zinc stimulates the formation of the heme part of haemoglobin.

- **Vitamins:** Folate and vitamin B_{12} serve as coenzymes that enable the production of DNA. Consequently, both are necessary for the production of new cells, including erythrocytes.

Disorders Associated:

- Anemia is characterised by a deficiency of healthy RBCs. This may occur owing to alterations in the cell or its components, such as haemoglobin.

- Spherocytosis is a disorder in which the body produces aberrant RBCs that are rounder and more spherical than a typical RBC's healthy disc shape. This renders the blood cells more fragile and susceptible to rupture. Hemolytic anaemia is a kind of spherocytosis. It is inherited, transmitted from parent to kid by genetic variations.

- Thalassemia impairs the body's capacity to manufacture haemoglobin and red blood cells (RBCs). As a result, a person will normally have fewer healthy RBCs. Thalassemia is a genetic disorder transmitted through the genes. There are several forms of thalassemia, depending on the characteristics that parents pass on to their offspring.

- Polycythemia, also known as erythrocytosis, is a disorder characterised by an elevated RBC count. The excess blood cells can thicken the blood and impede blood flow, which might raise the risk of various health complications.

Normal Constituents of Urine

Urine is a liquid waste of the body that is secreted by the kidneys during urination and excreted through the urethra. The majority of urine's natural chemical composition is water, but it also contains nitrogenous molecules like as urea, creatinine, and other metabolic waste substances. Other compounds may be expelled in urine if the glomeruli of the kidneys are damaged or infected, which might change the nephron's capacity to reabsorb or filter the various components of blood plasma. Urine is an aqueous solution composed of higher than 95 percent water and, in order of decreasing concentration, the following constituents:

- Urea 9.3 g/L.
- Chloride 1.87 g/L.
- Sodium 1.17 g/L.
- Potassium 0.750 g/L and
- 0.660 g/L for creatinine.

Other ions, inorganic and organic substances dissolved (proteins, hormones, metabolites). Several disorders can cause anomalous components to be discharged in urine or abnormal features to be found in urine. The most prevalent kinds of anomalous urine include:

- **Proteinuria** - The presence of protein in the urine, usually caused by leaking or damaged glomeruli.
- **Oliguria** – An unusually tiny volume of urine, typically caused by shock or kidney injury.
- **Polyuria** refers to an excessively high volume of urine, which is frequently induced by diabetes.
- **Dysuria**—Painful or unpleasant urination, typically caused by urinary tract infections.
- **Hematuria** is the presence of red blood cells in the urine as a result of an illness or injury.
- **Glycosuria** is the presence of glucose in the urine as a result of excessive plasma glucose in diabetes, beyond the amount that can be reabsorbed in the proximal convoluted tubule.

Unusual Components in the Urine

Proteins: Proteinuria (albuminuria) is the abnormal concentration of albumin and globulin in the urine. Normal basic tests are unable to identify the tiny amounts of protein (10-150 mg) present in normal urine. Pathologically, urine contains several proteins, including serum albumin, serum globulin, haemoglobin, mucus, proteose, and Bence-Jones proteins. Proteinuria is noticeable in glomerulonephritis. Neph-rotic syndrome is characterised by a significant proteinuria. Proteinuria increases as the severity of the renal lesion increases. Heavy metals, such as mercury, arsenic, or bismuth, can also contaminate the renal tubules due to pro-teinuria.

Glucose: Normal people excrete between 16 and 300 mg of sugar daily, which is difficult to detect with a simple test. When this amount or more is discovered in the urine, it is considered glycosuria.

Ketone bodies: In a typical 24-hour period, fewer than 1 mg of ketone bodies are eliminated in the urine. In hunger, diabetes mellitus, pregnancy, ether anaesthesia, and various forms of alkalosis, an increased number of ketone bodies are excreted in urine. Many animals may develop ketonuria as a result of excessive fat metabolism. In acidosis accompanied by ketosis, a larger quantity of ammonia is expelled.

Bilirubin and Bile salts: In situations of obstructive or hepatic jaundice, bilirubin is discovered in the urine. The excretion of bile salts is associated with bilirubinuria. During some phases of liver illness, bile salts may be discharged in urine without bile pigment. Traces of bilirubin without bile salts are eliminated in urine with severe hemolysis.

Blood: In addition to its presence in nephritis, blood is discharged in the urine during a kidney or urinary tract lesion. Free haemoglobin is also seen in urine following rapid hemolysis, such as in black water fever (a malarial consequence) or after severe burns.

Urobilinogen: In severe hemolysis, such as in hemolytic jaundice or pernicious anaemia, a portion of the bile pigment produced by haemoglobin breakdown is expelled in the urine as urobilinogen. When urine is exposed to air, colourless urobilinogen is converted into urobilin. This causes the urine to be orange-colored.

Porphyrins: Coprophyrins are generally eliminated in urine at a rate of 50-250 mg each day. Coproporphyria is excreted more when certain liver disorders are present. The urine of porphyria patients contains a higher concentration of coproporphyrins than normal.

Question Bank from Previous Years' Examination

Short Answers

1. What are monosaccharides? Give two examples.
2. Give one example each of di-, tri- and tetra-saccharides.
3. What are polysaccharides?
4. How will you test starch from iodine?
5. What are the structural and functional units of proteins?
6. Name six amino acids.
7. What is xanthoproteic test?
8. What is a biuret test?
9. How will you test for lipids?
10. What is denaturation and renaturation of proteins?
11. Define energy rich compounds with examples.
12. Write four differences between DNA and RNA.
13. Give the structures of any two essential fatty acids.
14. What is denaturation and renaturation of proteins?
15. Enumerate the role of following minerals in our body:
    1. Calcium   2. Iodine   3. Sodium   4. Zinc   5. Potassium.

    (a) Explain the properties of water (b) Explain the following terms:
    1. Osteomalecia   2. Goiter   3. Pellagra   4. Beri-Beri.
16. Mention the importance of Biochemistry.
17. How are amino acids classified?
18. What do you understand about the secondary structure of proteins?
19. Glucose or sucrose are soluble in water, but cyclohexane or benzene (simple six-membered ring compounds) are insoluble. Explain.
20. Write the structure of the product obtained when glucose is oxidised with nitric acid.
21. Give one example of each- Monosaccharide, disaccharide and polysaccharide.
22. Describe what you understand by primary structure and secondary structure of proteins.
23. Differentiate between fibrous proteins and globular proteins. What is meant by the denaturation of a protein?
24. What are the types of lipids? Discuss its classification.
25. What are proteins? Discuss its classification.
26. Write the inhibitors of ETC.

27. Define nucleosides and nucleotides.
28. Mention the bases of DNA and RNA
29. Write the biological functions of proteins.
30. Name the bile salts and give their significance.
31. Define the following as related to proteins:
    (i) Peptide linkage
    (ii) Primary structure
    (iii) Denaturation

Long Answers

1. (a) Write the structural and functional differences between DNA and RNA.

   (b) Name two starch components.
2. What is glycogen? How is it different from starch?
3. (i) Which one of the following is a disaccharide:
       starch, maltose, fructose, glucose?

   (ii) What is the difference between acidic and basic amino acids?

   (iii) Write the name of the linkage joining two nucleotides.
4. What is biochemistry?
5. Define carbohydrates classify them with example and their biological significance.
6. Explain glycogen storage disease.
7. Write the catabolism of purine Nucleotides.
8. Define genetic code and give its salient futures.
9. Explain the following terms:
    (i) gluconeogenesis
    (ii) Glycolysis
    (iii) Glycogenesis.

    (a) Discuss tricarboxylic acid cycle (Kreb cycle) and give its importance.

    (b) Write short notes on any two:
        (i) Glycogen storage disease
        (ii) Genetic disease
        (iii) Electron transport system.

10. (a) What are enzymes? Classify them giving suitable example for each class.

    (b) Describe the factors affecting enzyme reaction.

    (c) Write a note on enzyme inhibitors.

11. (a) What are proteins? Classify them. Write a note on quality protein.

    (b) What are biological functions of protein?

    (c) Give qualitative tests for protein.

12. (a) Define the term vitamin and classify them.

    (b) Enumerate coenzyme forms of water-soluble vitamins

    (c) Give biochemical functions of vitamin A and vitamin D.

13. Define and classify carbohydrates. Give chemical tests for monosaccharides.

    (a) Explain the following:

        1. Heparin
        2. Mutarotation
        3. Starch
        4. Diabetes mellitus.

14. (a) Discuss beta-oxidation of unsaturated fatty acid.

    (b) Enlist the abnormal constituents of urine and give their significance.

    (c) Give the major functions of Platelets.

15. Write short notes on any four:

        1. Optical isomerism
        2. Glucose tolerance test
        3. Role of Carnitine
        4. Lipid storage disease
        5. Insulin and its role.

16. (a) What are proteins? Classify them. Write a note on quality protein

    (b) What are biological functions of protein?

17. (a) Define and classify carbohydrates. Give chemical tests for monosaccharides.

    (b) Explain the following:

        1. Heparin
        2. Mutarotation
        3. Starch
        4. Diabetes mellitus

18. What are lipids? What are the functions of lipids in our body?

    (a) Write chemical tests for lipids.

    (b) Write note on:
        1. Phospholipids
        2. Glycolipids
        3. Lipoproteins

19. Define the term vitamin and classify them.

    (a) Enumerate coenzyme forms of water-soluble vitamins with their biochemical role.

    (b) Give biochemical functions of vitamin A and vitamin D.

20. 1. Enumerate the role of the following minerals in our body:
        (a) Calcium
        (b) Iodine
        (c) Sodium
        (d) Zinc
        (e) Potassium

    2. Explain the properties of water.

    3. Explain the following terms:
        (a) Osteomalecia
        (b) Goiter
        (c) Pellagra
        (d) Beri-beri

21. (a) Define the term vitamin and classify them.

    (b) Enumerate coenzyme forms of water-soluble vitamins with their biochemical role.

22. (a) What are enzymes? Classify them giving suitable example for each class.

    (b) Describe the factors effecting enzyme reaction.

    (c) Write a note on enzyme inhibitors.

23. (a) What are enzymes? Classify them giving suitable example for each class.

    (b) Describe the factors affecting enzyme reaction.

    (c) Write a note on enzyme inhibitors.

24. (a) Discuss beta-oxidation of unsaturated fatty acid.

    (b) Enlist the abnormal constituents of urine and give their significance.

    (c) Give the major functions of platelets.

25. Write short notes on any four:
    (a) Optical isomerism
    (b) Glucose tolerance test
    (c) Role of carnitine
    (d) lipid storage disease
    (e) Insulin and its role
    (f) ATP
26. (a) What are proteins? Classify them with examples. Describe two tests for proteins.
    (b) Explain β-oxidation of fatty acids.
    (c) Write a note on disorders associated with lipid metabolism.
27. (a) Define and classify carbohydrates with examples. Describe Molisch test for carbohydrates.
    (b) Write a note on disorders associated with carbohydrate metabolism.
    (c) Write a note on fat soluble vitamins.
28. (a) Define and classify lipids with examples. Add a note on function.
    (b) Write a note on water metabolism and its significance.
    (c) Write a note on blood and its constituents.
29. (a) Write normal and abnormal constituents of urine. Also, give their significance.
    (b) Write a note on diagnostic importance of enzymes.
    (c) Comment on gluconeogenesis.
30. (a) Explain glycolysis in details with energetics.
    (b) Write a note on mutarotation and inversion of sucrose.
    (c) What is biochemistry? Discuss its importance in pharmacy.